Getting Ready for Your Nursing Degree

PEARSON

At Pearson, we take learning personally. Our courses and resources are available as books, online and via multi-lingual packages, helping people learn whatever, wherever and however they choose.

We work with leading authors to develop the strongest learning experiences, bringing cutting-edge thinking and best learning practice to a global market. We craft our print and digital resources to do more to help learners not only understand their content, but to see it in action and apply what they learn, whether studying or at work.

Pearson is the world's leading learning company. Our portfolio includes Penguin, Dorling Kindersley, the Financial Times and our educational business, Pearson International. We are also a leading provider of electronic learning programmes and of test development, processing and scoring services to educational institutions, corporations and professional bodies around the world.

Every day our work helps learning flourish, and wherever learning flourishes, so do people.

To learn more please visit us at: www.pearson.com/uk

Getting Ready for Your Nursing Degree

The studySMART guide to learning at university

Victoria Boyd

Stephanie McKendry

PEARSON

Harlow, England • London • New York • Boston • San Francisco • Toronto
Sydney • Tokyo • Singapore • Hong Kong • Seoul • Taipei • New Delhi
Cape Town • Madrid • Mexico City • Amsterdam • Munich • Paris • Milan

Pearson Education Limited
Edinburgh Gate
Harlow
Essex CM20 2JE
England

and Associated Companies throughout the world

Visit us on the World Wide Web at:
www.pearsoned.co.uk

First published in Great Britain in 2012

© Pearson Education Limited 2012

ISBN 978-0-273-75089-5

British Library Cataloguing-in-Publication Data
A catalogue record for this book is available from the British Library

Library of Congress Cataloguing-in-Publication Data
Boyd, Victoria.
  Getting ready for your nursing degree : the study SMART guide to learning at university /
Victoria Boyd and Stephanie McKendry. -- 1st ed.
    p. ; cm.
  Includes bibliographical references and index.
  ISBN 978-0-273-75089-5 (pbk.)
  I. McKendry, Stephanie. II. Title.
  [DNLM: 1. Education, Nursing. 2. Learning. 3. Test Taking Skills. 4. Writing. WY 18]

  610.73071'1--dc23
                            2012002314

10 9 8 7 6 5 4 3 2 1
16 15 14 13 12

Typeset in 9.5/13.5pt Interstate Light by 3
Printed and bound in Great Britain by Henry Ling Ltd., at the Dorset Press, Dorchester, Dorset

Contents

6 Getting ready for the essay writing process

7 Getting ready for exams

Supporting resources

Visit **www.pearsoned.co.uk/boyd** to find valuable **online resources**

Companion Website for students

- Multiple choice quizzes
- Interactive practice activities
- Video and audio clips
- Assessment and revision planning templates to download

Preface

Whether you are already at university, are considering undertaking training within the NHS, or are just thinking about joining the healthcare profession, this book will help you prepare for studying.

More and more people are thinking about a career in nursing or healthcare, people who may never have wanted to be a student or seen themselves as very academic. But don't be put off by the fact that nursing is taught at university level. Just as, with practice, anyone can learn a practical skill such as changing a dressing, we believe anyone can learn the academic skills needed for university. This book will provide you with tasks and activities to support you in developing into an independent learner ready for university work.

The more you can work on your skills before or immediately on joining your programme, the quicker you will adjust to the course. This is true whether you are moving straight from school or college or have been away from education for some time. This book looks at all aspects of university work in a straightforward way, providing advice, examples and activities designed to help you get the most from classes, research and assessments. It is designed with nursing students in mind and is tailored towards the skills you will need not only for your course but for your career as a nurse.

Not just your average student

Studying nursing at university is different from learning any other subject. For a start, half of your time will be spent on placement: in a ward, community setting or other clinical area. You'll have lectures and theory to learn, but you'll also quickly be in the real world, applying what you've learned and caring for real people. The minute you enrol you are considered a healthcare professional and have to abide by the Nursing and Midwifery Council (NMC) Code. Try asking that of a sociology student or someone on a physics degree!

In other words, your life will be complicated:

- You will have to manage your time and balance lots of commitments (part-time work, placement shifts, assessment deadlines, social life).
- You may have to learn in new ways (lectures, tutorials, in clinical environments, in groups).
- You have to produce different kinds of work (essays, clinical documents, demonstrations of clinical skills).

So, to succeed, you will have to learn all of the theory, all of the clinical skills, and adjust to life in two, potentially, new environments (university and placement). It sounds difficult, but don't panic. If you are confident in your academic skills and you know the way you work best, you'll be able to do all of the other learning. That's where this book comes in.

What's in the book?

We've organised the content of the book to introduce academic skills in the order in which you're likely to need them.

- **Chapter 1** gets you to think about your past learning and how you can adapt your existing skills for life on a nursing degree. *Is a lack of confidence holding you back? Do negative experiences in the past still affect your beliefs about yourself and your abilities?*
- **Chapter 2** looks at studying at university. It covers what will be expected of you, what types of skills you'll need, as well as other things you need to think about, like your family and work commitments. *Universities use their own special language sometimes – we'll help you translate.*
- **Chapter 3** introduces the strategies and skills you'll need in class. *How do you concentrate for a full hour's lecture and come away with notes that will be useful? What on earth is expected of you in a problem-based learning (PBL) seminar?*
- **Chapter 4** is all about reading: finding information, understanding it and deciding what to use and what to discard. Nursing is an evidence based profession – you need to be able to get hold of and evaluate that evidence. *How do you know which resources to trust?*

- By **Chapter 5**, you'll have been to class, done the reading, and now you need to write something. It outlines the building blocks of academic writing – conventions, tone, and the dos and the don'ts. *You might have written essays before, but did they include references and up-to-date evidence for EVERYTHING you say?*

- **Chapter 6** is more of an in-depth look at essays in particular: how you go from being given the question and the hand-in date to submitting the final piece of writing. It covers planning, structure and looks at common mistakes to help you avoid some obvious pitfalls. *Does your essay present your reader with a logical argument? Do all of your sub-topics link together in a clear order?*

- **Chapter 7** recognises that assessments at university aren't just about essays. There are exams and numeracy tests, for example, and they require slightly different skills. Some people prefer essays, some people prefer exams, but you really need to be pretty good at all of them as they're skills you'll need in the workplace, once you're a nurse. This chapter looks at how to revise and tackle university exams. *How will you know what to revise? How will you divide up your time during the exam?*

- **Chapter 8** focuses on other types of assessment. In particular it explains and gives advice on reflective assessments, presentations and group work. *Do you know the distinctive features of reflective writing? Where will it fit in to your future practice?*

How to use the book

The chapters build on one another and take you through the skills as you work towards your first assessment, but they also all stand alone. So if your main concern is writing, for example, you can go straight to Chapters 5 and 6.

The book can be used before you start your programme, or even if you are thinking about applying to study nursing. That way, you'll have worked on your skills beforehand. *Getting Ready for Your Nursing Degree* will also be useful at any time within your first year, so you can practise note-taking while at a lecture, etc. But, equally, it never does any harm to review your academic skills at any point in the degree, so if you are in your second year and really want to work on your research skills, this book will be a handy companion.

Our advice on getting ready

If you only have time to do five things before you really get stuck in to your degree, we would recommend the following:

1. Read this book. Complete the activities and have a look at the additional features on the companion website.

2. Regularly read a nursing newspaper (such as the *Nursing Standard* or the *Nursing Times*). You could subscribe, or your big local library is likely to hold copies. This will help familiarise you with current issues and nursing language.

3. Keep a diary or learning journal. Record what work you do, how successful you were and other details. This will help you see your study habits. When are your energy levels at their highest? When is it pointless to even try to do some reading?

4. Look at your university's website, and find out as much as you can about what support is available to you.

5. Gather information about your degree. Is there anything specific you can do to prepare, such as reading the introductory textbook?

Publisher's acknowledgements

We are grateful to the following for permission to reproduce copyright material:

Figures
Figure 4.2 from *Journal of Clinical Nursing*, 20 (2011), Blackwell Publishing Ltd.; Figure 5.5 from www.nursingtimes.net, Nursing Times.

Screenshots
Screenshot 4.3 from EBSCO CINAHL Database.

In some instances we have been unable to trace the owners of copyright material, and we would appreciate any information that would enable us to do so.

Photos
The publisher would like to thank the following for their kind permission to reproduce their photographs:

Glasgow Caledonian University: Angus Forbes p. 99; **Department of Health: p.** 69

Cover images: *Front:* **Alamy Images**

Every effort has been made to trace the copyright holders and we apologise in advance for any unintentional omissions. We would be pleased to insert the appropriate acknowledgement in any subsequent edition of this publication.

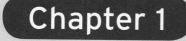

Chapter 1

Taking the obs

'Starting my nursing degree was one of the scariest things I've ever done. It was like entering an alien universe. I hadn't been in a classroom for 20 years let alone a lecture theatre. But, after some initial panicking, I soon realised it was one of the best decisions I've made'.

Third-year child nursing student

LEARNING OUTCOMES

By the end of this chapter you should be able to:

- Discuss in what ways your feelings and memories of education affect you now

- Evaluate your current skills and plan ways in which they could be adapted for use at university

- Understand and translate university/academic language

Introduction

This chapter is all about you: the way your previous educational experiences continue to affect you, the role that confidence can play in being a successful learner, and the wealth of skills you already have that will prove useful at university.

The role of confidence and your past experiences

Ready for take-off?

When starting any new journey, such as a new course and career, it's natural to feel excited or nervous (or both), but research has proven that how positively you approach a task can have an impact on how successful you are. Think about it – if too many of the little voices in your head are telling you that you can't do it, that's bound to have an effect.

So, make a bit of a space for yourself before we get down to the academic skills. How are you feeling? What's behind those nerves or that feeling of excitement?

ACTIVITY 1.1: ANYTHING TO DECLARE?

1. **List five words or phrases that describe how you feel about studying for a nursing degree. Are you anxious, over the moon or bored?**

....

....

....

2. **Write down one thing that you are really excited about or that you hope to get from your degree.**

....

....

....

3. Now write down one thing that worries you about your studies.

....

....

....

Turn to the feedback section at the end of this chapter to read our comments.

Any baggage to check in?

In many cases, the way that we feel about a particular thing is influenced by our past experiences of it. So when joining a new course, you're obviously going to be affected by how you've learned before, even if you haven't realised it yet.

It could be from school, college or a course that you reluctantly went on for work, but we all have baggage. Everyone has had a teacher who has made them feel that they could achieve anything: the maths teacher who went over fractions with you, using their own sandwiches, until you got it; the family member who knew you would pass your driving test and gave you the confidence to go for it. But similarly, there are those experiences that have had a negative impact, and they're often stronger: the swimming instructor who shouted at you; the other maths teacher who seemed to think there was something wrong with you because it took you a bit longer to understand fractions. All of these experiences create messages for us, and sometimes we still listen to them too strongly.

You're a completely different person today, and you needn't be stuck in a cycle. You're motivated, you're beginning a new course and there's going to be lots of support available. The reason that this book exists is that we firmly believe that academic skills, like any other, take time and practice to develop. Some people are more academic than others; their strengths are in writing, for example, but anyone can learn to produce a strong essay.

ACTIVITY 1.2: YOUR PREVIOUS EXPERIENCES OF LEARNING

1. Think of some really good experiences of learning in the past. What made them so enjoyable and effective? How did you feel? What message did you take from them, and what have they helped you to do today?

....

....

....

2. Now think of a time where learning wasn't quite so straight-forward. Did it give you negative feelings? If so, did they affect your confidence, and more importantly, do they continue to?

....

....

....

Turn to the feedback section at the end of the chapter to read our comments.

Recalling these memories will give you an opportunity to think about where your strengths lie and where you might need a bit of development.

Any nervous flyers?

Most people have pretty concrete ideas about their skills, attitudes, and abilities. So they take these beliefs with them when beginning a new degree. The psychologist Carol Dweck refers to these as 'self theories' and believes they can have a big impact on learning and motivation. She suggests that students tend to hold one of two views about intelligence:

1. An entity theory of intelligence

Some people think that your level of intelligence is fixed. You are simply born with a certain amount of it and can't do anything to change that. So, for example, you might believe that your sister is the smart one in the family, whereas you have no academic abilities whatsoever. The problem with this theory of intelligence is that it can stop people from putting in any effort – what's the point if you don't think it will make any difference? Students who hold this view of themselves can struggle to stay motivated or may not complete assessments. They can feel quite helpless because it seems like they have no control over anything.

2. An incremental theory of intelligence

Another view is that intelligence or ability is malleable, i.e. it can change. So, just like riding a bike, you may not be able to do it the first time you try, but the more you practise, the better you get. Students who hold this latter view are more likely to put in effort to master a particular skill or complete an assessment. They believe that their effort will have an effect, will produce a reward, like a good mark or personal satisfaction.

As you can imagine, there is some evidence to suggest that if you believe the entity theory, this can have a negative effect on your academic performance, especially if you lack confidence in your abilities. We believe in the incremental theory and that's basically what this book is about. If you put in the effort and practise you can develop strong academic skills.

If you want to know more about motivation and theories of intelligence and self, the main text to read is Dweck, C. S. (1999). *Self-Theories: Their Role in Motivation, Personality, and Development*. Philadelphia, PA: The Psychology Press. There are also lots of websites so a quick internet search will give you a good start.

What's your view of intelligence? Which theory makes most sense to you?

> ### A note on positive thinking
> Sports coaches put great emphasis on the power of a positive mental attitude. Athletes are encouraged to visualise crossing the finishing line in first place or scoring the winning goal. Research suggests this can have an effect on performance – if you imagine you are going to win, it can help you to do so.

▶

You may not buy this. Such visualisations may not suit your learning style and we certainly aren't asking you to change your beliefs. However, it is worth taking into consideration. Can you see yourself as a registered nurse? Do you believe you have put the work in to pass the exam? At the very least, have a think about the impact of negative feelings. In our experience, those students who honestly believe they can't write a good essay rarely find the motivation to put in the effort.

Confidence, effort and ability – two points of view

Student

At school it always took me ages to understand things. Everyone else would race ahead. So I decided education wasn't my thing. But I've always wanted to be a nurse, to care for people, and now that I'm older and more confident I'm not going to let a thing like uni get in my way.

In my first year, a lot of my friends seemed to leave everything to the last minute. It looked like they put in very little effort, but passed easily. Whereas I spent hours in the library and at home trying to get my head around everything. I've realised that it does take me a long time to research and write an essay. But I know I'm great at planning my time and making sure I meet the deadline. In fact, all that effort is really beginning to pay off. Now I'm in third year and I've got used to the skills you need, I'm not only passing – I'm passing well. It doesn't matter that it takes me longer than others. I get there and I understand my stuff when I do.

> **Tutor**
>
> It's often pretty easy to tell how much effort a student has put in to a piece of work. Someone could be a really skilled writer, or have lots of creative ideas but if they haven't put the hours in, they won't do well. University work requires lots and lots of reading and research. You have to spend time putting it all together, demonstrating your understanding and making sure you fully answer the question. There are no shortcuts.

Evaluating your current skills

You may be new to university, you may be new to healthcare, but you're not a blank slate. You have a wealth of skills and experiences. These can be used to help you in your degree. You might also have some bad habits, but there are ways to recognise and work around these. All of your skills, strengths, aptitudes – your history – can be transferred and adapted to university.

ACTIVITY 1.3: EVALUATING YOUR CURRENT SKILLS

Write a list of the things you're really good at, and think about what that means about your skills. How can you link these with preparing for university life?

I'm a great ...	This means ...	Skill for university?	Examples
Host	I know what my friends like. I'm good at organising things in advance and keeping everyone up-to-date.	Researching. Planning and organisation. Communication.	

Now do the same for something you know you're not very good at. Can you think of any solutions?

I tend to muck up ...	This means ...	Skill for university?	Examples
Getting to a new place on time.	I never leave enough time for the journey and often miss buses.	Find out how long journey is (research). Leave enough time (organisation). Stick to the plan (discipline).	

Turn to the feedback section at the end of this chapter to read our comments.

You might not feel that your experiences are particularly relevant, but have a look at the following two examples:

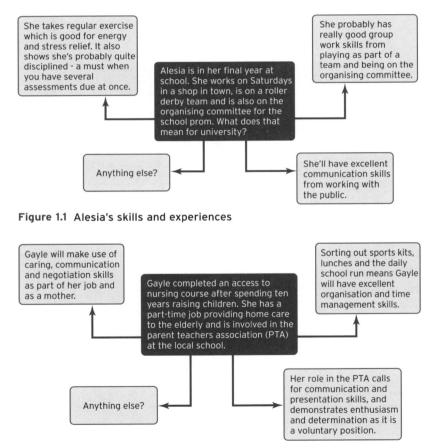

Figure 1.1 Alesia's skills and experiences

Figure 1.2 Gayle's skills and experiences

ACTIVITY 1.4: MAPPING YOUR SKILLS

Now, write a brief statement about your life and which skills you use. Can these be transferred?

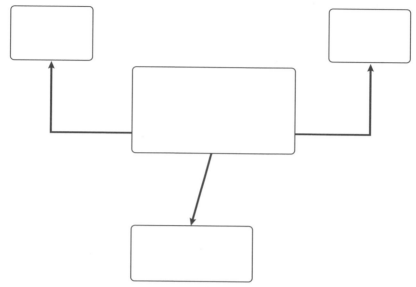

Figure 1.3 Your skills and experiences

Turn to the feedback section at the end of this chapter to read our comments.

Hopefully you've now thought about your previous experiences and whether any of them are holding you back. You've seen how important confidence (or a lack of it) can be, and that you have a bucket load of skills at your finger tips.

Translating university language

One thing you need to be aware of is that universities can seem like foreign lands - countries with their own language and customs - and nobody's given you a map and phrasebook. Don't let this panic you - finding your way is really just a matter of learning the language and asking the locals for help.

A note on why all the latin

So why is matriculation called matriculation and not just plain old registration, for example?

1 A lot of terminology used in universities is historical. It's about preserving tradition.

2 People who work in universities tend to have worked there for a long time. They know the ins and outs and sometimes forget that students are just passing through and may not. This isn't very fair.

3 The language used in academia has to be precise and clear (see, we're at it now: *Academia* = the world of university!). Academic debates may cross languages and subject disciplines, and all participants need to understand what the others mean. This can be confusing and takes a bit of getting used to, but once you've learned that language you can use it.

It's easy to have your head swimming after a few weeks with all this new university language AND healthcare related terms. Try to keep calm. Take a note of and then look up anything that you've never come across before. You won't be the only one in the class wondering what PDP, the NMC or the WHO is!

A quick phrasebook

Here are some of the words and phrases you're likely to come across at university. If there are others you don't understand, don't be afraid to ask for clarification, or look them up.

Bibliography	A list of all the books, journal papers and other resources you have used as evidence within a written assessment.
eLearning	You'll learn in lots of different environments at university: classroom, lecture theatre, skills lab. Sometimes it might just be you at a computer, completing a series of activities or taking part in a discussion board. This is referred to as eLearning. Just to confuse you, it might also be called blended learning or online learning.
Essay	This is a formal piece of written assessment. You may be expected to answer a particular question, evaluate a subject or theory, or make a case for one side of an argument. Word lengths vary but are not usually less than 1500 words. You will need to learn the conventions of academic writing and how to structure essays to be successful.
Lecture	A large class where a lecturer does most of the talking. It usually lasts one hour with a presentation on a set theme. It provides an overview of the topic which students should then supplement with additional reading. Notes may be given out in advance or made available online but it's essential to attend and take your own notes.
Matriculation	This is where you enrol for your programme, sort out your fees, get your student ID card. You usually need to do it every year of your degree.
Mentor	This is the person who will support you while you are on placement. They are qualified practitioners who have an interest in education and wish to help new students. They will assess your skills and help you record your clinical learning. There may also be student mentors who help you get used to life at university.
Module	Most courses are divided into a series of different units. These are usually called modules. At any one point you will be studying at least a couple of them.
PBL (problem-based learning)	A form of learning in which you're given a scenario or problem, and as part of a group conduct research and report back. There is limited (if any) involvement from staff.
Placement	A period of time spent in the clinical area where you will be engaged in active learning. You will work alongside, and learn from, nursing and other healthcare staff. This is where you get to put the theory into practice.

Plagiarism	This is a form of cheating. It can be deliberate but often students do it without meaning to, simply because they do not reference their work properly. Basically, it means passing off someone else's work as your own – another student, work from a book, journal, website or wherever.
Portfolio	An ongoing, written record of your learning. Lots of courses have these, but in nursing it is a key element, and will include your placement experiences and evidence of achieving clinical proficiencies.
Programme	There's lots of confusion about this term as individuals call it different things. This is your course, your degree ... the thing you're studying for three or four years.
Semester/ Trimester/Term	The academic year will be split up into different sections with holidays in between. It varies from university to university. Make sure you know the university dates, exam times and holidays. There's usually a calendar of academic dates on the university website that will give you this information.
Seminar/Tutorial	These are smaller classes in which you'll be expected to actively join in. You'll prepare beforehand and often speak during the session.
Tutor/Facilitator/ Lecturer	Academic staff play many different roles. Sometimes they will talk at you for an hour, sometimes they'll be leading small discussion groups, sometimes they won't talk at all. It's up to you to find out which of these roles staff are performing. They're never just your teachers.
VLE (virtual learning environment)	An online space where teaching materials are made available. Different universities use different systems (e.g. Blackboard, WebCT, Moodle). You may use discussion boards and even submit essays through it.

Go to our companion website to try an online activity on translating healthcare jargon.

What to take from this chapter

- Emotion plays a strong role in learning, so it's a good idea to recognise how you feel about things when beginning a course. Is a previous experience holding you back?
- You have loads of skills already from different aspects of your life. You can adapt many of these for university.

● Don't get caught out if it seems like you don't understand things at first. Universities have their own language, and it can take a while to learn. Just because things might be new to you doesn't mean you shouldn't be at university.

Reflective questions

At the end of each chapter, we've included a few reflective questions. They are a brilliant way to apply what you've read to your own learning, circumstances and experiences.

1. Are you ready to do the best you can at this course? Have you addressed any anxieties? Are you mentally prepared?

....

....

....

2. What are you best at? How can you play to your strengths when at university?

....

....

....

3. Do you know the terms your institution uses? Could you translate as many of these as possible before you join your programme?

....

....

....

Further support

Your university will have a form of confidential student counselling or wellbeing service. If you do have any concerns about your confidence, look for a link on your university website or students' homepage for further information.

Feedback

Activity 1.1: Anything to declare?

1. What does this description say about your state of readiness? Is it going to help you succeed? Is it perfectly understandable and unavoidable? Do you need to take any action?

2. Our students tend to say that they are most excited about becoming a nurse, joining a profession and gaining a qualification. This desire, even inspiration, can be a great help in keeping you motivated through the harder times. Unlike other subjects, your degree has an end goal and, hopefully, a lifelong career. Use that ambition to drive you on.

3. In our experience, students say they are worried about being prepared enough for placement learning and the workload involved. They also share lots of concerns about themselves – insecurities like, 'Am I good enough?', 'Do I deserve to be here?', 'Will I be able to write essays?'

4. We start each year asking our students to anonymously write down one hope and one fear – 99 times out of 100 these dreams and worries are exactly the same among the whole group. So take comfort that you are not alone in having doubts (if you do). It's completely understandable when you've made such a big decision and commitment.

Activity 1.2: Your previous experiences of learning

Are you embarking on this new programme in the right frame of mind? Are you spending too much time listening to the voices that hold you back? If previous experiences are affecting your confidence, what are you going to do about it?

Activity 1.3: Evaluating your current skills

This should give you a good idea of your current position. What are your strengths and weaknesses? What action might you need to take to address bad habits and develop good ones? We cover this in a bit more detail in the next chapter.

Activity 1.4: Mapping your skills

Your answer here will be completely unique to you. The point is that you have lots of skills.

Chapter 2

Learning to learn: life as a student nurse

'It took me until my second year to figure out that it's just as important to be able to search databases for journal articles as it is to accurately monitor blood pressure if you're going to pass.'

Third-year adult nursing student

LEARNING OUTCOMES

By the end of this chapter you should be able to:

- Describe the characteristics of an independent learner at university
- List the academic skills you need at university, and evaluate your current strengths and weaknesses
- Identify aspects of your personal circumstances that can both support and potentially impede your success

Introduction

The purpose of this chapter is to demonstrate that you have to learn how to learn at university. It's a completely different environment from school, college or the workplace, so as well as the clinical skills and the theory (content), you also have to develop learning skills (researching, referencing, academic writing).

The student nurse experience

Siobhan has recently completed her Bachelor of Nursing degree at Glasgow Caledonian University. We've worked with her throughout the three years of her course and asked what advice she would give to new students.

My life as a student nurse

Siobhan Fairhurst
When I was asked to write this piece, I thought it would be best to highlight the reality of nursing and the hardships and sacrifices you may need to make. Now, don't get me wrong, there are many of those, and they will all differ for each of you. For some it will be time you sacrifice – time with your family and loved ones. For others it will be money – moving from well-paid jobs to follow that career change. And for others, it may just be your sanity from time to time!

However, on reflection, what I really want to say about being a student nurse is, 'Go for it!' With all your heart, or as much as you can donate. You really do get out what you put in, and you have to put in a lot. That sounds very sentimental, but this is YOUR vocation, that YOU have chosen … so do it justice.

I'm not saying I haven't had those 'what am I doing?' moments, wondering if I'm good enough or if the reality is too different from the books. But each time I have a connection with a patient and hear them say that I have made a difference to them, sometimes simply with a smile or a five-minute conversation, I know I'm home and where

I should be. If you want the classic 'student experience' and to party for three years ... you're in the wrong place!

Different people choose nursing for different reasons, whether its job security and money, status and respect, or to see the world. Whatever the reason, you will get the best experiences and satisfaction by being motivated by passion and enthusiasm for being a nurse and doing the best you can for others. That best starts now, from day one, in how you approach training and commitment to your studies. Be committed and this will make the journey far easier than resenting the workload or being beaten by alternative attitudes you meet in university or out in practice. Being a student nurse is a bumpy ride, full of ups and downs. Just as well you're strong and the kind of person who wants to make a difference and be part of something bigger.

Now, we are all different. Some are great with essays. Some the practical stuff. But you need to develop skills in both. You will always find support and help, but you have to ask. Make yourself known to study support teams and lecturers. I did, and it meant that those educating me knew me well and where I needed help. They could see the effort I was making and how I thought things through. If you are offered academic support, TAKE IT! And early too, so you can get ahead of the game and be less stressed. Plus, if you don't have a positive experience or are having issues on placement, staff will know who you are and be able to support you better. A nursing degree will help you mature to levels you never thought possible and you will be dealing with things you never thought yourself capable of. Be open to that, and you will see yourself grow in knowledge and skill before your very eyes.

Above all, be organised, enthusiastic and don't be afraid to give a little of yourself to each person you meet. Love you or not, you will have been true to yourself, maintained your own high standards and brought the best care you could to the people that matter most ... the patients. A mentor of mine said something to me once that has stayed with me since. Each patient is someone's mum, dad, granny, etc. So see the person, and not the problem!

Finally, and last but not least ... the study of nursing and the human body is fascinating, and advances in healthcare will astound you. So, go boldly where no student nurse has gone before ... within NMC regulations of course. And HAVE FUN!!!

Success at university – becoming an independent learner

In the same way that you need to adjust to a new language and vocabulary at university, there are lots of new responsibilities that come with being a student nurse. At school and college, teachers may have noticed if you weren't there or if you didn't understand something. In a lecture theatre of 500, that just can't happen.

Put bluntly, you chose the course, so it's up to you to attend classes and put the work in. There's lots of support available for you, but the difference is that you have to ask for it.

As usual, university has its own set of terms for these responsibilities. You may hear people talk about being an independent learner, a self-directed learner, an adult learner or an autonomous learner – these all mean the same thing.

Attributes of an independent learner

1. Takes **responsibility** for their learning.

Debbie is struggling to understand what is expected of her at university. She has made an appointment to speak with her tutor and is attending skills workshops.

Rosemary has failed an assessment and doesn't know why. She was given a written explanation, but doesn't understand it, and hasn't asked anyone for clarification.

2. Manages their time effectively.

At the start of term, Steve finds out assessment hand-in dates and writes them on his wall-planner. He plans everything else around them.

Ruth has spent two hours on three separate buses to get to university, only to discover she's got her days mixed up – the tutorials are tomorrow.

3. Organises and **plans** their learning, setting themselves targets and working out how to reach them.

Judith has a presentation to plan and deliver. She attends a class in using PowerPoint and gets some leaflets on improving her public speaking skills.

Chris has three essays due next week and hasn't started any of them. He plans to ask for extensions.

4. Recognises that they have to **learn how to learn** at university.

Richard is just about to go into his third year. He knows that he's supposed to take a critical approach in assessments, so has asked his tutor what that means.

Amy has been at university for a few months, and still struggles to get anything from lectures. It seems like everyone else is coping brilliantly.

5. Asks questions and is curious about subjects.

Adam always makes sure he prepares for tutorials by reading in advance. He can then join in discussions about the topic and learn from other students.

Unless Jean is specifically told to look at something by her tutor, she doesn't. She feels cheated if a topic she doesn't expect is covered in an exam.

6. Solves problems.

Karen has failed several exams before. This time around she has arranged to speak to a tutor about her nerves and has planned her revision well in advance.

Gerry falls ill and misses lots of classes. He receives a letter from the university about his absence, but doesn't get in touch because he's worried.

7. Is **motivated** and **enthusiastic** about their learning and makes an effort to understand why their programme covers the material it does.

Ross doesn't see the relevance of studying sociology on his course, but he tries to link it to nursing and it becomes a lot clearer after his community placement.

Martha thinks you should only study nursing. She has decided psychology is boring and stops going to classes.

What skills do you need for university?

To become an independent learner, and succeed on your programme, there's a set of skills that you require. Some you may have, but need to advance to a university level; others will be entirely new. In the activity that follows, we have provided a list and definitions of the skills we think each student nurse should have as part of their toolkit.

ACTIVITY 2.1: PATIENT PROFILE

Name: _____

Temperature	_____ °C
Pulse	_____ bpm
BP	_____/_____
Resp	_____
Pain Score	_____

With patient	y/n
Valuables listed	y/n
No medication required	y/n
Taken home	y/n
Details:	

Patient can:	Self-diagnosis (1 – poor, 5 – excellent)	Evidence of skill	Care plan
Example – note-taking	4	*Took good notes during practice lecture and was able to retrieve information afterwards*	*Practise taking notes from TV a couple of times before programme begins*
Independent learning (understand the nature of learning at university)			

Patient can:	Self-diagnosis (1 – poor, 5 – excellent)	Evidence of skill	Care plan
Note-taking (can take effective notes in lectures and from books and journals)			
Finding resources (find paper and electronic resources using library and web)			
Critical reading (choose and use appropriate resources for university level – evaluate rather than just describe content)			
Academic writing (write with an appropriate style and structure for university)			
Academic referencing (provide evidence in written work through in-text citations and a reference list)			
Working in a group (complete tasks effectively as a member of a group)			
Presentation skills (plan and deliver a strong individual or group presentation)			
Numeracy (demonstrate appropriate levels of numeracy for safe practice)			
Planning and organisation (ability to manage time, organise plans of activities and stick to them)			

Patient can:	Self-diagnosis (1 – poor, 5 – excellent)	Evidence of skill	Care plan
ICT skills (use computers to access information and complete assessments)			

Figure 2.1 **The patient profile**

Remember, we provide comments or feedback on all activities at the end of each chapter.

Go to our companion website for a blank copy of the patient profile.

Myths and misunderstandings about university

We find that people often come to university with similar ideas of what to expect. Unfortunately, these are sometimes wrong and can cause needless anxiety. The most common misunderstandings include:

Myth 1: You do not have a full timetable

Yes, you do. If you're on a full-time programme, you should be working a minimum of 35 hours a week on your studies. Whilst your classes may only take up ten hours each week, there's lots of independent work that you need to do to prepare for them and complete assessments. See the following examples:

The timetable in Figure 2.2 looks pretty empty, doesn't it? You could easily think that your Fridays are free.

	9-10	10-11	11-12	12-1	1-2	2-3	3-4	4-5	5-6
Monday	Tutorial	Lecture		Lecture		Lecture			
Tuesday		Biophysio Lecture		Lecture	Tutorial			Lecture	
Wednesday	Tutorial		Biophysio Tutorial						
Thursday	Clinical skills lab	Clinical skills lab	Clinical skills lab						
Friday									

Figure 2.2 A typical timetable of your classes

25

	9-10	10-11	11-12	12-1	1-2	2-3	3-4	4-5	5-6
Monday	Tutorial	Lecture	Go over lecture notes from last week	Lecture		Lecture	Go to library to read and prepare for tomorrow's tutorial presentation		
Tuesday	Find resources for essay	Biophysio Lecture		Lecture	Tutorial		Prepare for Biophysio tutorial and go over lecture notes		Attend academic writing workshop
Wednesday	Tutorial		Biophysio Tutorial			Fill in clinical skills log book for last week		Prepare for this week's clinical skills session	
Thursday	Clinical skills lab	Clinical skills lab	Clinical skills lab						
Friday	Read and take notes for essay								

Figure 2.3 Your timetable once you've added in study

	9-10	10-11	11-12	12-1	1-2	2-3	3-4	4-5	5-6
Monday	Tutorial	Lecture	Go over lecture notes from last week	Lecture	Lunch with Sue	Lecture	Go to library to read and prepare for tomorrow's tutorial presentation		
Tuesday	Find resources for essay	Biophysio Lecture		Lecture	Tutorial		Prepare for Biophysio tutorial and go over lecture notes		Attend academic writing workshop
Wednesday	Tutorial		Biophysio Tutorial	Aerobics		Fill in clinical skills log book for last week		Prepare for this week's clinical skills session	
Thursday	Clinical skills lab	Clinical skills lab	Clinical skills lab		Shift at work				
Friday	Read and take notes for essay			Childminding					

Figure 2.4 A typical timetable when you add your life

You need to prepare for each of those classes and there'll be lots of extra reading and coursework to be done. It's vital that you plan and find the time for those activities. No one else is going to tell you when to do them.

It's unlikely that there will be nothing else going on besides your university work. How are you going to fit everything in?

 Go to our companion website to try an online activity about managing your time at university.

Myth 2: You're supposed to be independent, so you shouldn't ask for support or help

Well, we'd be out of a job if you didn't. Students often think that tutors don't want them to ask questions or for clarification, but actually we do. It's far better to have a full understanding of a topic than to sit in silence because you're worried you'll look silly if you speak out. You'll also find that there are lots of support services at university, so if you're having financial problems, finding the library difficult to navigate or don't know how to reference, there'll be someone there to help. Learning independently doesn't mean learning in isolation.

Myth 3: You should already have all the skills you need

As we've already said, you have to learn how to learn at university. Why be there if you know it all already? Nobody expects you to be able to administer an intramuscular injection when you first start, so why should you be able to do a literature review? In addition, in each year of your degree more is expected of you, so you'll be constantly developing your skills.

Myth 4: Learning is more difficult when you get older

Rubbish. There is no evidence to suggest that mature or adult learners perform less well than younger students. If you've come straight from school, you have the advantage of being used to full-time study.

However, if you're returning to education as an adult, you have that wealth of life experience to draw on.

Myth 5: If you fail something, struggle or fall behind, there is no way of catching up

University isn't that harsh. There are always opportunities to re-take assessments. The really important thing is to speak to your tutors, and seek support if you are having problems. Don't fall too far behind without taking action. Approach tutors as soon as you think there may be a problem. They're much more likely to help than if you turn up at the last minute.

Myth 6: If you didn't enjoy school or past education experiences, you won't enjoy university

As we said in Chapter 1, there is evidence to suggest that holding on to those negative feelings about previous educational experience can affect your current performance. It can make people lose confidence and fail to ask for support or clarification when they need it.

University is very different from all other learning and you are now a different person. There is no reason to think your experiences will be the same as before. You have chosen to be there for a start!

Myth 7: Everybody else is finding it really easy, it's just me having problems

Trust us, it may seem the case. But it isn't!

Your life as a student – are you ready?

Hopefully, by this point in the book, you:

- have considered your feelings and experiences and thought about the impact they might have on your current confidence and learning

- know what is expected of you in terms of becoming an independent learner at university
- have a good idea of what academic skills you'll need and know where your strengths and weaknesses lie.

So, is there anything else you need to think about before getting stuck in to the skills stuff? There are other things that can hold you back or are potential barriers to successful study. It's worth thinking about these beforehand. What can and can't you control? In what ways have you come unstuck in the past?

Overcoming hurdles – knowing where they are before you have to jump them

The types of barriers you may face (the things that could stop you doing as well as you hope) fall into three categories:

1. **You** - your likes, dislikes, habits, patterns of behaviour. These all have an effect. Some are helpful, such as your sheer determination to complete a task when you're up against it. Others less so, like a complete inability to ignore a text message.

2. **Your life** - your family, friends, job, charity work etc. These all have an impact on your time, motivation, mood, energy and even finances. This, inevitably, has a knock-on effect on your studies.

3. **The institution** – the university, degree, module etc. There may be things concerning the institution that stop you from getting things done. All copies of a particular book being out of the library, for example.

Knowing how these three categories may affect you personally, the stuff you can work around and the things you can change, will help you start off on the right foot.

Confidence
The stuff we've already talked about in terms of the little voices holding you back

Learning preferences
How do you like to learn? Are you a very visual person or do you learn more effectively when someone tells you information? How can you incorporate this knowledge into your study plans?

Your bad habits
Are you a procrastinator (put things off to the last minute)? Are you really forgetful? Are you always late? What can you do to get round these tendencies?

Your hurdles

Organisation and planning
Work out when, where and how you work best. Are you a morning person? Do you prefer silence or working to music? Get to know yourself and use that knowledge when planning for university work.

Your distractions
They are everywhere: email, TV, text messages, phone calls, music. Which ones are you particularly unable to ignore? Is there a way to manage them (e.g. switch off your web connection so you can't browse when writing)

Health and wellbeing
Look after yourself. When are you going to exercise and relax? Do you have health considerations to take into account?

Academic likes and dislikes
You will prefer some topics to others. How will you stop yourself drifting off for those you find less interesting? How will you overcome your fear of maths for example?

Figure 2.5 Your own hurdles

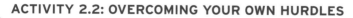

ACTIVITY 2.2: OVERCOMING YOUR OWN HURDLES

Think about your personality and consider the examples above. What is likely to help and hinder you? What can you do about it? Be honest.

The issue	The impact	The solution

Turn to the feedback section at the end of this chapter to read our comments.

A note on procrastination

Procrastination is very common and can strike at any time. People do it because they are intimidated by the sheer scale of the task, focus too much on one aspect of the work at the expense of the rest, or simply don't want to do it. Others are perfectionists, so they never quite complete anything.

There are lots of techniques you can use to avoid procrastinating. Break that scary task into smaller activities, each will feel a lot more manageable then. Do the hardest thing first; it gets it out of the way. If you feel you really need to stop, try going for another 15 minutes. Often that's enough to make real progress or even get you completely over the lull in energy. And most importantly, decide whether you are studying or not. Don't waste time on the space in between - so don't sit with your books taking nothing in and don't go to the cinema but feel really guilty. One or the other.

ACTIVITY 2.3: OVERCOMING YOUR LIFE HURDLES

Think about your circumstances and consider the examples below. Are any of them relevant to you and will they affect your studies? What can you do about it, if anything? Might there be any changes over the course of your degree?

The issue	The impact	The solution

Turn to the feedback section at the end of this chapter to read our comments.

Caring commitments
Kids, nieces, nephews, parents, uncles, sisters, neighbours. Quite rightly, these responsibilities will still take up a significant amount of your time. How will you fit your studies around them? How will you let them know when you need to be left alone to work?

Part-time or voluntary work
Most students have some form of work on top of their studies. This can be really great experience but how will you manage your time? Can you cope with the hours?

Relationships
Friends and partners will be a great source of support to you and will be able to help you relax. But they can sometimes make demands on your time that affect your studies. How will you manage this?

Social life
You need time off for good behaviour and you're going to be meeting lots of new people. But you have to get the balance right.

Life hurdles

Finances
This is a category in its own right because it is always such a worry for people. Have you budgeted? Do you need to look for other sources of income? Are these concerns stopping you studying?

Life admin
This is all the stuff you have to get done for your life to run smoothly – pay bills, sort out insurance, buy birthday presents, all the unseen things that take up time. Can you organise this better? Could you delegate?

Housework
It's got to be done. When will you hoover, shop for food etc.? It's really common to use housework as an excuse not to study. Do you have a tendency to iron when you should really be in the library?

Careers/employability
You are on the degree because you want to become a great nurse. The planning for this starts now. Should you be gaining other skills (such as leadership)? Are you so worried about the future it's affecting your studies?

Figure 2.6 Your life hurdles

Staff availability
Tutors don't live in boxes waiting for the moment you need to discuss the essay question. They are usually only too happy to help, but find out when they're available and make an appointment in advance. You might get more out of the meeting if you have a specific idea of the kind of support you require.

Access to IT facilities
Universities have invested a great deal in IT facilities, but they're not always going to be perfect. So think about potential problems, plan ahead and know where to go for help. The network might go down as you are trying to submit an assessment or you may not find a free computer when you need one.

Timetabling
You will have very little, if any, control over this. The university has to arrange 1000s of classes for 1000s of students so it's always complex. Once you know your timetable think about travel time, childcare, how to maximise study time in between classes.

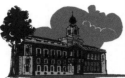

Institutional hurdles

Study facilities
You are likely to spend at least some of your study time on campus. Whilst there'll be some great facilities, others may be problematic. Perhaps a lecture theatre has a dodgy screen or a supposed quiet study area is actually really noisy. Find ways around these annoyances. Sit at the front or go home to study, for example.

Rules and regulations
The university will have procedures and ways of doing things that you need to follow. For example you will submit assessments in a certain form and certain way. Or you may have to pay fees or library fines by a specific time. Life can become needlessly complicated if you fail to get this right, so find out what's expected as soon as you can.

Student representation
A lot of institutional barriers are simply part of life and can't be helped. However, if you feel it is an issue that can be resolved there are ways of having your voice heard - a students' association or class rep system for example.

Figure 2.7 Your institutional hurdles

ACTIVITY 2.4: OVERCOMING YOUR INSTITUTIONAL HURDLES

These are likely to be specific to your institution and you may not be able to anticipate many yet. So you might like to come back to this exercise once you're familiar with your university and the way it works.

The issue	The impact	The solution

Turn to the feedback section at the end of this chapter to read our comments.

Hopefully you've now had a chance to think about your past, your strengths, your current circumstances and what's expected of you. Now it's time to move on to the university skills.

What to take from this chapter

- Be proactive and ask for help when you need it. It's your degree, your learning and your effort. Ultimately, it's you who has the career at the end of it all.

- You have to learn how to learn at university. There are specific academic skills that you'll need, and now is the time to start developing them.

- Part of becoming an independent learner is becoming aware of habits, tendencies, preferences and personal circumstances. There are things you can change about your life, and things that you can't. But even with the latter, it's possible to find ways to work around them.

Reflective questions

1. What do **you** need to do to become an independent learner?

....

....

....

2. Do you have an achievable action plan to develop your academic skills?

....

....

....

3. Pick one thing about yourself that you know has had a negative impact on previous study, and that you hope to change.

....

....

....

Further support

You need to manage your whole life as a student nurse. Things such as your finances, accommodation, childcare, any additional learning needs should all be considered. Ideally, you can sort these things out before beginning your degree, but if not, then pretty quickly on joining. Speak to your university or look at their website for local details. The following organisations may also be of use:

National Union of Students (NUS): http://www.nus.org.uk/

Nursing and Midwifery Council (NMC) students page: http://www.nmc-uk.org/Students/

Royal College of Nursing (RCN) students community: http://www.rcn.org.uk/development/students

In our experience, the maths and science content of a nursing degree can cause quite a lot of anxiety among new students. Reading up can help:

Foss, M. and Farine, T. (2007). *Science and Nursing and Healthcare*, Pearson Education Ltd.

Garret, L., Clarke, A. and Shihab, P. (2011). *Skills for Nursing and Healthcare Students: Study Skills, Maths and Science*, Pearson Education Ltd.

Reid-Searle, K. *et al.* (2009). *Student Nurse Maths and Medications Survival Guide*, Pearson Education Ltd.

Shihab, P. (2010). *Numeracy in Nursing and Healthcare: Calculations and Practice*, Pearson Education Ltd.

Feedback

Activity 2.1: Patient profile

Hopefully this activity has given you a good overview of the skills you require. This book takes you through the majority of them and helps you practise and develop. It's probably a good idea to assess your skill level once you've finished the book, and then at regular intervals through your degree.

 We've provided a blank copy of the patient profile on our companion website to allow you to do this.

Activity 2.2: Overcoming your own hurdles

There are possibly behaviours, habits and self-beliefs that you know have such a negative impact on you it's worth trying to change them. But often this is really difficult, if not impossible, to do. Mostly, it's about recognising your tendencies and adapting them or using them to your advantage. So, if your weakness is trashy TV, we aren't saying that you need to go cold turkey. How about rewarding yourself with an entire evening of reality TV's finest once you've handed in your assessment? A little self-awareness can go a long way.

Activity 2.3: Overcoming your life hurdles

We are not saying that your studies should be your absolute, number one priority. It's about recognising all of the parts of your life and finding the right balance. So, if you have children, for example, the Saturday evening take-away and TV ritual might be unmoveable. You just need to plan around that and enjoy the time you do have together. Of course you can't plan for everything. People become ill. The unexpected happens. At least if you are organised you can have contingency arrangements or maybe anticipate problems. So if your friend has a crisis the week before your essay is due, if you have started well in advance, you can probably afford to spend a couple of evenings dispensing the hankies and chocolate.

Activity 2.4: Overcoming your institutional hurdles

There are some barriers you simply can't control. Whilst this might be frustrating, the important thing is to anticipate them and find a way around them. The experience helps you to become independent and forward thinking. So if you miss a deadline because the computer packed in, learn from that for next time round and submit a few days in advance.

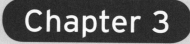

Chapter 3

Getting ready for classes

'My absolute favourite thing at university is when we have a brilliant lecturer. We have some amazing speakers who I could listen to for hours. Whenever I'm feeling low they're a great source of inspiration.'

Second-year mental health nursing student

LEARNING OUTCOMES

By the end of this chapter you should be able to:

- Describe the features of the different classes you'll attend at university

- Develop your own note-taking and active listening strategy for lectures

- Create an action plan to help you prepare for and participate in tutorials and placement learning

Introduction

This chapter provides an overview of the different classes that you'll participate in at university and the skills that you'll need for them. It concentrates on the three main places in which you'll learn: the lecture theatre, tutorials and placement.

Classes at university

Why attend classes?

You'll find that your timetable is a mixture of different classes. You'll be studying different subjects within your degree – biology, sociology, physiology and psychology, for example, as well as nursing. But even within the same module you'll learn in a variety of ways and environments. This is good news, as it keeps things interesting.

Obviously, there will be the odd occasion where you have to miss a class due to illness etc., but it's really important you get into good attendance habits. Classes give you the opportunity to:

- meet other people
- focus solely on your studies for a period of time
- hear experts talk about their subject.

While you could borrow notes from a friend, listen to an online recording or podcast of a lecture, or download the presentation, it is not the same as attending. There's simply no substitute for being there in person.

Types of classes

Classes that you may come across include:

- large-group lectures
- smaller-group tutorials or seminars
- practical learning in clinical skills labs

- one-to-one support tutorials
- problem-based learning (PBL) groups.

(Please see the phrasebook in Chapter 1 for a fuller definition).

Some classes require different skills from others, but as you can see from the table below they all interact. So, the skills that you are developing will be of use to you time and again.

	Lectures	Tutorials	Placement
Active listening	✓		
	You need to actively make sense of what you're hearing.		
Concentration	✓		
	You need to stay engaged when someone is talking for up to an hour.		
Confidence		✓	✓
		You have to speak in discussions and give presentations.	You must make the most of the learning opportunities and seek out as many as possible.
Communication		✓	✓
		You need to make yourself understood.	You have to interact with patients and fellow professionals.
Note-taking	✓		✓
	You need to capture the information for use, perhaps six months later.		You'll write handover notes, take histories and complete documentation.

	Lectures	Tutorials	Placement
Participation		✓	✓
		You have to bring along research and ideas and be prepared to discuss them.	You need to get as involved as possible in order to gain from placement experiences.
Preparation	✓	✓	✓
	You'll read up on the topic beforehand and ensure you print off any slides the lecturer makes available.	You must know what is expected of you in a particular tutorial and have done the work beforehand.	You will research the placement area so you know what to expect.
Questioning		✓	✓
		You should use the opportunity to ask questions and clarify issues with staff and fellow students.	You'll need to ask questions constantly to make the most of the experience.

Figure 3.1 Skills required for different classes

Lectures

Picture the scene. You're in a room of 500 students. People are arriving late. There's someone behind you eating crisps. The student beside you is texting, loudly. The lecture is about the NMC Code – you know it's important and that it will come up in the exam, but you don't know anything about it at this stage. You've never had this lecturer before and you're finding it quite hard to understand their accent. ARRRRGH!

Don't panic. We both remember those first few weeks at university. They were exhausting. Your hand aches. You're not too sure you've actually learned anything yet. But before you know it, you're completely used to attending lectures.

So what can you do to get the most out of them?

- Check if there's a version of the lecture slides available online, typically on your university's VLE (virtual learning environment). If so, print out and read them to familiarise yourself with the topic and terms. At the very least you should know the lecture title and could do a bit of background reading.

- Make sure you arrive in plenty of time and choose a good seat near the front. Apart from giving yourself time to get your notes organised, pens out and getting the best view you can, you also know the lecturer can see you. Psychologically, what could help improve your concentration more than that?

- Have everything you need with you: pen, spare pen, laptop, phone on silent. That way you're committed to giving the lecture your full attention for that space of time.

- Block out distractions as best you can.

- Take notes, even if you have a handout. Ideally, your notes will be completely individual and will still make sense to you in six months' time.

If you do all of this, hopefully you'll have gained a good understanding of the lecture topic and written useful notes for the future.

Active listening

ACTIVITY 3.1: HEARING VS LISTENING

If you think about it, hearing and listening are two different things. You can hear lots of sounds at once. Stop and think – what can you hear just now?

....

....

....

Traffic? Typing? Music? People in the corridor outside?
Now think, what are you actually listening to? We can really only concentrate on one sound fully.

What are some of the things that you know distract you when you're trying to listen? What can you do to block them out?

....

....

....

As always, turn to the feedback section at the end of the chapter to read our comments.

We've all got a brother, daughter, husband or sister that you know fine well can hear you, but is not listening. There's a big difference between the two.

Listening is a skill. To listen to a lecture, understand it and make notes takes time, practice and a great deal of effort. It's a really steep learning curve when you first start university. The thing that makes it challenging is that this type of listening is *active*, rather than *passive*.

A note on the need to be active

You might conscientiously attend every lecture. You print the slides because you feel you can listen better if you don't take notes. Things may start off quite well, but you soon find some of the lecturers talk quickly and you begin to panic. Other times, you decide the topic is uninteresting and your mind wanders. If it's hot in the lecture theatre or the class is taking place towards the end of the day, you may even struggle to stay awake. The problem here is that you aren't getting anything from attending the classes. Lectures are a brilliant way of receiving lots of information from experts who have done all the hard work for you, but only if you're actively listening.

It's worth noting at this point that if you have a hearing impairment, that doesn't necessarily mean that you can't develop active listening techniques or alternative strategies to ensure you keep active. Talk to your university's disability services about techniques that might work for you and the support that is available.

Suggested exercises for active listening

Try some of these activities to develop your active listening technique. It might be best to experiment with just one per lecture, but test them out and see what works for you.

- Focus on what you are thinking about during lectures. Are you actually mentally writing a shopping list, remembering last night's TV or planning your holiday?

- Summarise issues in your head. Put the arguments, concepts or theories in your own words. This helps you to test whether you understand them and maintains your concentration.

- Reflect on your reaction to information - is it new or surprising? Where does it fit with what you know already?

- Relate the information to other sources you have consulted - other lectures, textbooks, journals. You understand and retain information a lot better if you make links and can fit it together with your previous knowledge.

- Ask yourself, where does the lecture content fit into nursing and healthcare practice? What does it mean for the nurse?

The important thing is to become very self-aware. Recognise when you are daydreaming and fix it. If you realise that you've lost your place, don't worry. Just begin listening and note-taking from then on. You can always do more reading to fill in the gaps later.

If you know that you're prone to drifting off, what about setting a vibrate reminder on your phone to go off in your pocket at regular intervals? It might just be enough to bring your focus back. Just try not to scream with fright!

Features of the lecture

Something that may help, too, is that lectures tend to follow a similar pattern, and you'll get to recognise this. Every lecturer is unique with their own style of presentation, slide layout, mannerisms, speed and skill, but there's a general structure to the lecture itself.

First five minutes	**What's happening?** Lectures tend to start with an overview that indicates the content. Sometimes you're even given learning outcomes (what you are supposed to have learned from the lecture) This is also the point at which any important announcements might be made.
	Challenges: People may still be coming in. It's noisy. You might not be in the right frame of mind yet. You may have even had to rush to make it to the class on time.
Main body of the lecture	**What's happening?** This is where you get all the detail. Pay particular attention to repetition of phrases or concepts and use of examples. It's likely that these are the key points that you are to take away.
	Challenges: Maintaining concentration can be difficult. You must follow the structure and flow of what can be a lengthy argument, recognising the important points, blocking out background noise and getting used to the lecturer's style.
Last five minutes	**What's happening?** Lectures will end with a summary of the content. Ideally, you're told the key 'take home messages'. Sometimes you'll be pointed to further reading and references.
	Challenges: Lecturers are often really rushing to fit in all the detail. You may be really tired, and you probably have some place to be shortly. There may also be a lot of noise from the people who are eager to leave and those waiting to enter the room.

Figure 3.2 Timeline of the lecture

Be aware of and prepared for the different phases of the lecture.

Getting the most from lectures

- **Prepare in advance.** Background reading will help to familiarise you with key concepts and phrases. Know what the lecture will be about at the very least. It's all part of being an independent learner.

- **Keep checking whether you are concentrating.** We know we keep saying this, but it's just so easy to lose concentration.

- **Don't become emotionally involved with the content.** It will stop you listening to the next section.

- **Try not to dismiss a subject as uninteresting.** It may not be immediately obvious where a particular topic fits into your course, but it wouldn't be included if it wasn't relevant!

Note-taking

Why take notes?

You can often get the lecture slides beforehand or there's even possibly a podcast or audio recording of the lecture, so why take notes?

1. 'I've got the handout, so I'll just listen instead.' There's a lot of additional information given out in the lecture that won't be on the slides. They are a bare minimum, a good starting point, but you need to fill in the detail.

   For example, a lecturer may talk you through this diagram for ten minutes, whereas on the handout you just have the picture.

The Retina

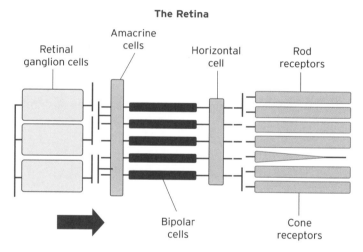

Figure 3.3 An example lecture slide (Source: Dr Ross Goutcher)

2. 'I know this stuff already. It's been covered in school and college, and it's all just common sense anyway.' You can't use common sense in an assessment – you have to provide evidence for everything, so it's important to capture detail accurately. You may have covered the topic before, but you'll be expected to have a deeper understanding at university.

3. 'I don't know what the important points are.' Spend time preparing beforehand. Do some background reading. Learn to anticipate points, the use of repetition and your lecturer's style.

4. 'I'll remember it.' Few people have a photographic memory, and your notes need to be useful to you in six months' time – perhaps even longer. It's well known that taking notes aids your understanding. You're having to process the information and put it into your own words. It also really helps you to concentrate on the topic.

5. 'I can't write quickly enough.' It takes time and practice to build up your stamina and develop the right type of note-taking technique for you.

6. 'I can't understand what the lecturer is talking about.' Prepare in advance. Make a note of the points you don't understand and speak to your tutor about anything that is unclear.

Note-taking techniques

There are a number of techniques that you can try out to find a style of note-taking that suits you:

1. Notes on VLE slides

Some lecturers will make slides available on your university's VLE before the lecture. This is useful as you can print a copy to take along that will give you the basic structure and content of the lecture. But remember, there will be lots more detail included in the lecture itself, so it's important to add your own notes, questions and ideas.

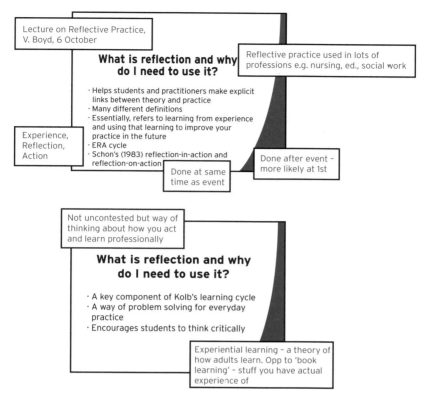

Figure 3.4 Example notes on lecture slide print-out

2. The Cornell system

The Cornell system works by dividing the page into three parts:

- The cue column: on the left-hand side of the page. Write down the main concepts, terminology, etc. here.

- The note-taking area: the main part of the page where you note as much detail as you can.

- The summary: a space at the bottom of the page which allows you to write, in full sentences, selected main points of the lecture.

Learning from experience and applying it to future practice	**Reflective Practice (V. Boyd, 6 October)**
	• Helps practitioners link theory to practice
	• Experience, Reflection, Action (ERA)
	• Schon (1983)
	    1. Reflection in action – at the time
	    2. Reflection on action – afterwards

Cyclical theory of adult learning through experience
Dif. models of reflection
	Kolb's experiential learning cycle (1984)
	  1. Concrete experimentation (event)
	  2. Reflective observation (personal thoughts on that event)
	  3. Abstract conceptualisation (relating to theory, why did this happen)
	  4. Active experimentation (test theory in practice. Apply learning)

All emphasise what happens next. What can be learned.	Gibbs 1988 • Series of q's to structure reflection. Leads through description, to analysis, action plan for future and on to next occurrence of event • Dynamic process – never stop reflecting or learning from it Johns 2000 Rolfe 2001

Numerous reflective models exist. Many of these are designed to help practitioners reflect upon and learn from their professional experiences. Based on Kolb's theory of experiential learning, professionals are encouraged to think about incidents and the feelings they provoke. They should also consider what they could do to improve their performance in a similar situation in the future.

Figure 3.5 Example of Cornell system notes

3. Mindmap

Many students prefer to learn visually, using a mindmap, linking ideas and concepts with images, colours and text. There are several software packages available to help you with this, but you can create mindmaps by hand. Start with the main concept in the middle, then move outwards, with different branches representing different topics, and lines and arrows showing how concepts are connected.

This can also be a great way to plan assessments or revise.

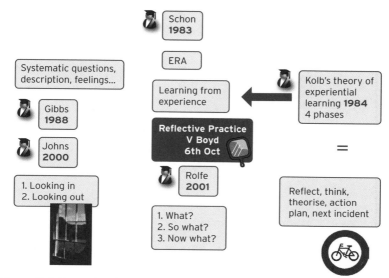

Figure 3.6 Example of notes using a mindmap

ACTIVITY 3.2: FINDING YOUR OWN NOTE-TAKING TECHNIQUE

Find a podcast or recording of a radio show to takes notes on (something with talking rather than music). Radio programmes are fast-paced with lots of content, and you don't get any visual clues, so it's purely about listening.

Take notes, without thinking too much about it, for about five minutes.

What do your notes look like? Do they make sense when you read them back to yourself? Would they still be useful a few months from now?

....

....

....

Now take another five minutes, and try the Cornell system. Ask yourself the same questions as above.

....

....

....

Finally, for another five minutes, try a mindmap.

....

....

....

Do you have a preference? If so, why?

Turn to the feedback section at the end of this chapter to read our comments.

Go to our companion website to watch some lectures and have a go at note-taking.

Tutorials and seminars

A tutorial or seminar involves a much smaller group than a lecture, with students expected to make a contribution to discussion. You'll find the terms tutorial and seminar are used interchangeably, but they basically mean the same thing.

The tutorial is a chance for you to consider a topic which has been covered in a lecture in more depth. It's also an opportunity to ask any questions which you may have noted down in the lecture or during your background reading. Before the tutorial, you're likely to be given the topic and a reading list of recommended books and journal papers. Though you don't have to consult all of these, it's important that you read widely to gather as many facts and perspectives as possible to give you a rounded picture of the subject.

Typically, a tutor will lead the discussion. On other occasions, a member of the class or a group will present on a tutorial topic, before a general discussion takes place. Everyone will take a turn at doing this.

Sometimes the entire group is set a problem and students have to decide among themselves how to analyse the subject and who will perform what role within the group. This is often referred to as problem-based learning (or PBL), and you are likely to meet it in some of your classes in the future.

A note on the three P's

We think that there are three key elements to getting the most from tutorials:

- **Preparation:** always do the work beforehand.

- **Participation:** make an effort to get involved.

- **Presentation:** practise and gain confidence in speaking and sharing your views with the group.

What makes a bad tutorial? A tutor's view

'One of the worst things that can happen to you as a member of academic staff is the painful tutorial: trying to generate some sort of interaction with ten stony-faced students for up to an hour. I've been with this group for three weeks and can't seem to get a word out of them. I don't know if they don't understand the topic, they're not doing the preparation, they're all really shy ... or they just hate me and each other. Nobody's learning anything here. I talk and talk but the only way we'll make progress is if we discuss these issues. I want to know who thinks what, what arguments they've been convinced by and how they think it fits into their future nursing career. This isn't a lecture – I'm not supposed to be teaching. I need the students to talk'.

Getting the most from tutorials

Sometimes it can be a bit intimidating talking in a group. But just try to remember that seminars and tutorials are an opportunity for you to improve and build on your knowledge – no one is trying to put you on the spot. If you prepare well for a seminar or tutorial session you will find them very rewarding and a useful source of revision materials. Here are some tips for preparing and contributing more fully.

- **Make sure you do as much as you can of the reading that has been allocated.** That way you will be more comfortable with the subject and armed with the knowledge to fully participate in discussion.

- **Note down any questions or comments that you might have to raise in class.** You can even practise these out loud at home beforehand to make sure you're confident with them.

- **Start small.** Even if you only say 'yes' or 'no' in response to a point that someone is making, you are still showing willingness to take part in discussion and that you are following what the class are talking about with interest.

- **Have a strategy for getting involved.** Raise some of the points that you wish to bring to the discussion by:
  - looking for a pause in the discussion
  - making eye contact with the tutor to let them know you have something to say
  - adopting confident body language
  - agreeing with what someone has said and adding your own thoughts
  - challenging what someone has said and providing reasons for your position (in a nice, polite way, of course!)
  - asking a question.

- **Get to know the other people in your class.** If you can, sit with someone who you feel relaxed with.

- **Remember, it isn't a test.** The tutorial is a chance for you to discuss your ideas in a supportive environment.

- **Take your time and speak slowly.** Try to talk confidently (even if you're not!).

- **Working in a group is a skill.** It will take some time and practice to develop.

Placement learning

The development of your skills, confidence and communication techniques will also be of great benefit on placement. You'll spend about 50 per cent of your time in one clinical setting or another: learning 'on the job', observing the professionals, asking questions and practising your clinical skills. You will work alongside mentors, members of staff who are there to provide support and education while you're in the practice setting. Just as with lectures and tutorials, there are various things that you can do to maximise your learning in this environment.

Getting the most from placement learning

- **Remember that your placement is a learning experience.** You are not expected to turn up on the first day with all of the skills and answers. You will learn while you are there, so ask lots of questions and get support if you need it.

- **Discuss any issues with your mentor.** Solution-orientated rather than problem-based discussions tend to be more productive, so have a clear idea of what the issue is and what kinds of support might help. Agree on goals and strategies. University staff will also be available for support if necessary.

- **Work on your time management.** Set yourself reminders if you lose focus, and work on concentration and motivation strategies. BUT ... don't lose confidence if you feel you are always being hurried along. This happens to everyone. We all tend to be slow at new tasks.

- **Read up on your area.** There's usually a little time before your placement to do some research. What's the nature of the setting? What patients, procedures and health issues are you likely to encounter?

Note-taking on placement

From an academic skills point of view, the main issue with placement learning is note-taking. At university, it's possible to use laptops or scribes. But on placement, strategies for note-taking will be purely pen and paper-based. This can be an adjustment for everybody, as we don't tend to write by hand very much any more. However, it can be a particular issue for students who have English as an additional language or an impairment on the dyslexia spectrum. Again, it's about having a clear understanding of what's expected of you and preparing in advance.

- Anticipate when you will take notes. Shift handovers? Any other times? Will other people need to understand them? Think about spelling, handwriting and redrafting.

- What is the vital information? You only need to note down the important details. Know what these are likely to be in advance. Practise quick ways of writing them – train your hands.

- Work on your listening skills. Learn to listen for the important information among everything else. If you always take details from the same speaker, recognise their style/accent/tone. Work on your concentration – are you listening or daydreaming? You'll have developed all this from attending lectures.

- Consider vocabulary issues. Throughout the course, develop vocabulary cards and lists to help you remember words and spellings. Have small cards to keep around you or put lists all over your house. Work on your vocabulary before placement. Think about words you will need for the particular clinical area. Any drugs names, for example? Add to vocabulary lists as you go. Look up spelling on placement if necessary.

- Think about abbreviations. Learn official abbreviations. You can develop your own, but only use them for personal notes. You will need to translate if someone else is to understand. Speak to your mentor if you don't understand any abbreviations.

- Create a pocket pack. Tools you can carry in your pocket to enhance your confidence. Vocab cards? Medical spell checker? Cover overlays? Checklists/grids? You can cut them to size to make them discreet.

- Develop checklists and grids and make copies beforehand. Think about issues you tend to have, things you sometimes forget or get wrong and include them in the list (see example in Figure 3.7).

Task	Done?
Checked drugs spelling?	
Signed everything?	
Legible to others?	
....	

Figure 3.7 An example placement checklist

The key, then, is to practise. You are learning a new skill. It will take time and patience to develop. Accept that you may need to work on your note-taking.

Go to our companion website to try an online activity on taking notes on placement.

What to take from this chapter

- Attend lectures and take notes. This is the most effective way to get hold of the knowledge that you need and retain it in a usable form for the future.

- Actively engage in tutorials. They're not a learning environment if nobody speaks.

- For any type of learning, the more you can prepare beforehand, the more you'll get out of it. This is true for lectures, tutorials and placement.

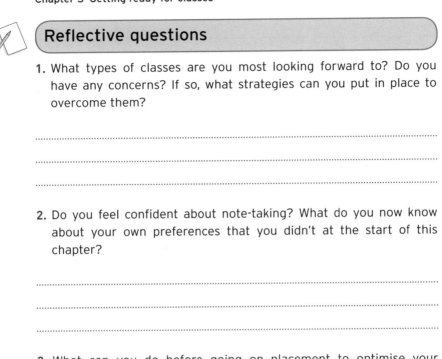

Reflective questions

1. What types of classes are you most looking forward to? Do you have any concerns? If so, what strategies can you put in place to overcome them?

....

....

....

2. Do you feel confident about note-taking? What do you now know about your own preferences that you didn't at the start of this chapter?

....

....

....

3. What can you do before going on placement to optimise your learning while there?

....

....

....

Further support

A lot of our students have found the following book really useful, especially when planning for placement:

Siviter, B. (2008). *The Student Nurse Handbook*, Balliere Tindall.

Feedback

Activity 3.1: Hearing vs listening

Your answers to this activity will be completely unique, depending on where you are. It might be worth trying a few times in different situations.

Activity 3.2: Finding your own note-taking techniques

It's surprising how tiring note-taking can be. The combination of active listening, concentration and writing with such intensity takes a bit of getting used to.

You may find that your own combination or adaptation of the suggested techniques suits you best.

Chapter 4

Getting ready to find resources

'At college we were always given the reading we needed by our tutor. It took me ages to realise that you have to go and find all this stuff for yourself at university. It was quite scary at first but then I realised how much freedom it gave me.'

First-year midwifery student

LEARNING OUTCOMES

By the end of this chapter you should be able to:

- Identify and locate different resources for use in university work
- Develop your own criteria (reading questions) to decide whether something is appropriate to use in academic work
- Decide on your own system for taking notes from resources

Introduction

In this chapter we'll talk you through the variety of resources you will use at university. We'll look at how to make the most of them, the stuff to avoid and how to make effective notes for use in assessments.

Why do I need to find resources?

So you've attended the lecture. Next week there's a tutorial on the same topic. How do you go about preparing for it? You will need to find resources in order to develop an in-depth knowledge of the subject area because you will be expected to discuss it. The lecture and the material provided by your tutor are only the introduction – a taster or general overview of the theme. As an independent learner, you are expected to go away and do lots more research on that topic. You'll find information, read and understand it, and then present your arguments within classes and assessments.

You also need to be able to find resources so that you can provide evidence for everything you say within your assessments. This is one of the key conventions or characteristics of academic writing. Your work at university must be balanced and objective. So you have to provide evidence or references for absolutely everything. Otherwise it will look like unsubstantiated opinion.

Compare the following statements:

- Poor people tend to be fatter than rich people.
- Richardson (2008) has suggested a link between low economic status and obesity. This is perhaps due to lack of access to education (Smith 2005).

The first statement provides no evidence to support the argument it makes. It appears opinionated, subjective and, perhaps, even preju- diced. The second statement makes the same link between the two factors (poverty and obesity), but does so by referring to an author and published evidence. It then goes on to consider explanations for that link. The first is not appropriate in an academic piece of writing; the second is.

Here are another two examples:

- Young children can find it very stressful to stay for extended periods in hospital. They may suffer homesickness and be unused to separation from their parents. This could have an impact on the outcome of their treatment.

- Separation anxiety is well documented among hospitalised children (James 2007). As a result, NICE (2008) recommend the use of family rooms wherever possible, and research has suggested that this can have a positive impact on treatment (McDonald 2001).

As a nursing student, you are on your way to becoming an evidence based practitioner. Your practice and professionalism will be underpinned by the best, most recent research. You will need to be able to find and understand that evidence, as well as all of the latest guidelines and current government policies. It isn't just about showing what you know; it is necessary in order to provide the best care you possibly can.

You will be given a reading list for each module (if you are not given one, ask). This contains recommended textbooks and journal papers. It's up to you to find them, and you'll be using much more than just the ones on the list.

In your university work, you *could* use pretty much anything: newspapers, TV programmes and discussion boards, for example, are all potentially useful and could be considered academic 'texts'. However, you have to have a valid academic reason for using them.

Gathering information and evidence on a particular topic is called searching the literature.

Types of resources

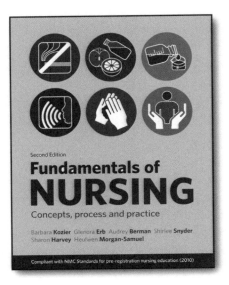

Figure 4.1 Textbook

Textbook

What it is: A general introduction to a subject (e.g. *An Introduction to Psychology for Nurses and Midwives* or *Essentials of Physiology.*)

Where to find: These will be available in your library as hard copies or, sometimes, eBooks.

When to use: They are probably the first place you'll turn to, to get a broad overview of a topic, to find definitions or to clarify your understanding of something. For example, if you need to provide a definition of autonomy in an assessment, you could consult a textbook on ethics in nursing to find a suitable one.

Positives: They tend to be written in an easy-to-understand style, often aimed at a specific year of study. They are sometimes even written by your lecturers and designed for your course. They are easy to come by in your library or bookshop.

Negatives: They are only introductions, a jumping off point that should lead you to more in-depth resources. They tend to become out of date quite quickly (it takes so long to write, edit and publish a big book like that, practice and research may already have moved on by the time it's on the shelves).

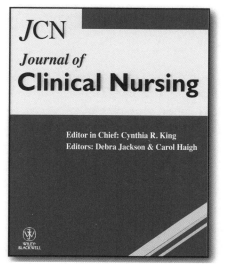

Figure 4.2 Journal cover

(Source: *Journal of Clinical Nursing*, Cynthia R. King (Ed), Copyright © 2011, Blackwell Publishing Ltd. Reproduced with permission of Blackwell Publishing Ltd.)

Journal paper/article

What it is: A journal or periodical is like a magazine on a specific topic (such as coronary healthcare, research in nursing or mental health issues in teenagers). The journal produces several issues per year, and each issue contains a number of papers (sometimes also called articles) all written by different people. Each paper will be broadly related to the overall theme but will be on a very specific topic within that.

So, if we were thinking about this in everyday terms: a journal is like a weekly magazine and a paper is like an article written by a celebrity columnist.

Where to find: Journals may be available in your library as paper copies. They often also have online versions which you can access and print out from home. Some journals are only available electronically.

When to use: Journal papers are a brilliant source of information. You will use them when you need in-depth knowledge for assessments. The sooner you become confident in finding and reading journal papers the better, since you need to move on from general textbooks relatively quickly. For example, you might be writing about oral health promotion. You could find a paper that specifically investigates the impact of a promotional campaign in primary schools in Wales and include the results in your essay.

Positives: Papers tend to involve research, so make recommendations for healthcare practice based on evidence. They are specific and tend to be fairly short, so you can gather a great deal of information quickly. They also have an abstract at the beginning. This is a 100–200 word description of the paper that allows you to quickly judge if it is going to be valuable to you. Journal issues are produced so regularly you can find very up-to-date information on the topic you are researching.

Negatives: It generally takes too long to simply browse through relevant journals to find papers. You need to know what you are looking for. You will search databases by putting in key terms in order

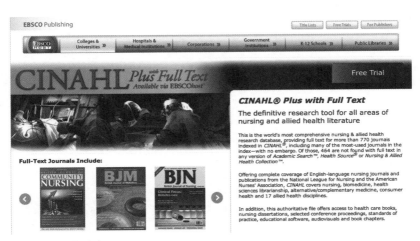

Figure 4.3 Database

to find out what has been published on a particular topic. This is a core academic skill and can take a little time and practice to master. Journal articles tend to be written using complex vocabulary and a dense writing style (the author is putting a huge amount of information into a very short space). They can be quite difficult to read at first. Again, a bit of patience and practice will help you here.

Database

What it is: These are search engines to find journal articles. You put in particular search criteria, such as key words, dates, authors' names, and the database provides you with a list of matches. There are lots of different databases. Some, such as CINAHL, AHMED and Medline, are particularly geared towards searching for UK nursing and healthcare information and papers.

Where to find: You will be given access to databases via your university's network (either from a campus computer or logging on to the university system from home). There is a skill to searching databases, but don't worry, there will be lots of support from your university – either time in class, advice from librarians or online guides. It's often a bit hit and miss at first. You try out some search terms on a database and get thousands and thousands of search results, so you tweak the terms and then get too few ... It's really a matter of perseverance.

When to use: You'll use databases whenever you need to gather resources for classes or assessments. Typically, you will have been given a topic. You come up with search terms for it (words that express the general or related meaning) and put them in to relevant databases. The results will provide you with the details of journal papers that have been published on that topic – you then access and read these. For example, you might be conducting research for a presentation on cancer pain. You could find suitable papers by searching databases using terms (words) such as 'cancer', 'oncology' and 'neoplasm' for the cancer element of your search, and 'pain', 'pain management' and 'pain assessment' for the pain aspect.

Positives: Databases search a lot of different journals at the same time, including all of their previous issues. You can limit searches so they only include papers published in the last three years, for example. Often it is possible to link directly from the database search results to the actual papers. This means you can sometimes conduct all of your research from your home computer with a few clicks of your mouse!

Negatives: Databases give you access to so many papers it can be difficult to filter through the results. It isn't as simple as searching on a library catalogue or an internet search engine and this can be offputting. You will need time and practice to use databases, but they are the best way of finding scholarly, appropriate resources.

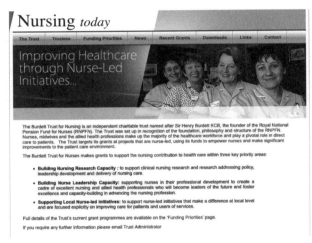

Figure 4.4 Website

Website

What it is: A group of pages published on the internet.

Where to find: The majority of campus computers are likely to have internet connections and you will be allowed access to websites for university-related work. Please bear in mind that your university will have a policy on the use of ICT (Information and Communication Technologies) facilities, so take care when accessing websites and make sure their content is appropriate.

When to use: Almost all government bodies, professional associations, journals and healthcare organisations have websites. So they are a great way to access up-to-date information and publications. For example, perhaps you are writing about public perceptions of health issues. You could use newspaper websites, health forums and the sites of pressure groups to investigate the range of opinion.

Positives: They provide instant, often free, access to information and resources. They can also provide a forum and voice to groups and individuals who may not otherwise be heard.

Negatives: Anyone can fairly easily publish on the internet. So you have to be cautious about which websites you visit. You should only be reading credible resources backed up by evidence. Does Bob's '101 reasons why I absolutely hate the NHS' page provide this?

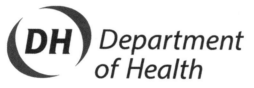

Figure 4.5 Government publication and legislation

Government publication and legislation

What it is: These might be from the Department of Health, the UK Government or other governments. Things like the Human Rights Act or mental health bills may inform your daily practice as a nurse.

Where to find: You may find paper copies in libraries or online versions on government websites.

When to use: They are excellent resources to use in assessments to demonstrate your understanding of important legal developments in healthcare. For example, you might refer to child protection legislation when discussing the role of the children's nurse in a community setting.

Positives: Used alongside journal articles. These resources show you are aware of the broader context in which your healthcare practice operates.

Negatives: They won't provide you with detail or explanation, and are often written in a legal language that can be tricky to understand.

Policy documents and guidelines

What it is: Lots of organisations don't just inform, they sometimes even regulate what you do. These include the NHS (National Health Service), NICE (National Institute for Health and Clinical Excellence), SIGN (Scottish Intercollegiate Guidelines Network), the NMC (Nursing and Midwifery Council) and the WHO (World Health Organisation).

Where to find: All organisations have websites and produce publications in print and electronic form.

When to use: When you want to talk about an aspect of practice. So, for example, if you were writing an essay on gaining a patient's consent before treatment, you may want to refer to the NMC Code, to show that it's a legal and professional obligation.

Positives: They show your awareness of professional responsibilities.

Negatives: It may not be as obvious how to reference some of these documents as it can be with other types of resources you'll use.

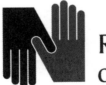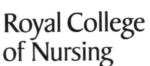

Figure 4.6 Other organisations

Other organisations

What it is: These might include charities (e.g. MIND, Macmillan), pressure groups (e.g. patients' rights organisations) and professional bodies (e.g. RCN or Royal College of Nursing).

Where to find: Really, you could use anything as a resource, including commercial companies, but you have to be very careful selecting what to include. It's important you have an academic justification for any choice you make.

When to use: When they provide credible and relevant information. For example, a piece of work on palliative care might be really enhanced by using research published by Macmillan.

Positives: They can be very focussed and specific. You get another perspective, perhaps one from a patient's point of view.

Negatives: You really need to think about bias and whether you can trust the evidence you wish to include.

How do I know I'm reading the right stuff?

One of the really good things about writing on a nursing degree is that you do get to include lots of different types of information in building your argument. But with a limited word count and limited time available, you need to be very selective and it's important that you develop ways of choosing appropriate information (inclusion criteria).

ACTIVITY 4.1: QUESTIONING THE EVIDENCE

You've come across this news article and wonder whether you could use it as evidence in an assessment.

A group of scientists at the University of Westmorland have discovered that bird song is a form of laughter, providing evidence that birds possess a sense of humour. Led by Professor

Rudolph McKay, the team used human psychology research to investigate finches' reaction to humorous stimuli.

The study, funded by the Avian Research Studies Executive, showed 20 birds video footage of cats falling over and recorded the ensuing bird song for analysis. 'The twittering reactions from the finches proved conclusively that birds share human beings' sense of humour – a fact that, until now, we had not considered', reported Professor McKay. 'We think that a sense of humour in the avian community is important as birds are collective beings, and may use laughter in conflict resolution.'

Until now, it was thought that bird song was largely intended to attract a mate or warn of danger, but this research suggests a much more sophisticated function. The US military are currently engaged in discussions with Professor McKay about whether this new knowledge can be used in intelligence operations.

Use the following questions in making your decision.

1. What claims do the researchers make?

....

....

....

2. What evidence do they use to substantiate these claims?

....

....

....

3. Are the claims rational, justified, convincing? Why?

....

....

....

4. Are there any logical problems?

....

....

....

5. Any other pertinent information?

....

....

....

6. What is your overall judgement on this research?

....

....

....

You can find our comments in the feedback section at the end of the chapter.

Reading questions

A good way of ensuring you are reading and including appropriate resources is to develop a reading checklist - a series of questions you ask yourself about any source of information or evidence. We've suggested some questions below:

Date	Notes
What is the date of publication?	
Does this affect the value of the text?	

Is it out of date? Any changes in legislation since it was written (e.g. research on smoking before/after the ban)?	
Author	**Notes**
Who wrote the text?	
Am I told anything about their background?	
What are their qualifications? Are they an authority on the subject?	
Are there any biases or vested interests I should be concerned about?	
Kind of publication	**Notes**
What kind of text is this – journal, book, website?	
Is it from a respectable source?	

Is it peer-reviewed? (Has it been reviewed by experts before publication?)	
Evidence	**Notes**
Has sufficient and relevant evidence been included to support the argument the author makes?	
Has the author shown a good understanding of the topic and other research in the area?	
Are any recommendations made and has the author related the evidence to healthcare?	
Relevance	**Notes**
Is the text on the right topic?	
Is it of suitable reliability for use in university work?	
Have I got time to read it?	

▶

Others (any other questions you should ask?)	Notes

Figure 4.7 Critical reading questions

A note on peer-reviewed papers

The best journals use a peer-review process to ensure the quality of the papers they publish. Each paper that is sent to the journal is evaluated by several experts in the field (a bit like university marking). These reviewers will decide if the paper has used a suitable research design or considered all of the important issues, for example. They inform the editors whether they believe the paper should be rejected, published or returned to the authors for correction.

You can work out whether a journal uses this process by looking at the 'information for authors' section of the website. This will tell you what an author can expect to happen when they submit their paper.

Always try to determine whether a paper has been through the peer-review process. It doesn't mean that you can accept everything it says as fact, but it does provide you with additional information to judge the contents.

Go to our companion website for a beginner's guide to reading a journal paper.

ACTIVITY 4.2: DECIDING ON THE SUITABILITY OF SOURCES

There's a lot of information available that at first glance can seem interesting and relevant, but that wouldn't necessarily be appropriate for use in academic work. The bird article is a good example of that.

Consider the following different sources of information. Many students use them in their university work. But should they? Would you?

Wikipedia

1. Is it suitable for university work?

....

2. What are the reasons behind your decision?

....

....

....

NHS24

1. Is it suitable for university work?

....

2. What are the reasons behind your decision?

....

....

....

Mumsnet

1. Is it suitable for university work?

....

2. What are the reasons behind your decision?

....

....

....

Nursing Standard or *Nursing Times*
1. Is it suitable for university work?

....

2. What are the reasons behind your decision?

....

....

....

Google
1. Is it suitable for university work?

....

2. What are the reasons behind your decision?

....

....

....

Turn to the feedback section at the end of this chapter to see our comments

Why take notes?

So you've searched the literature and found a selection of relevant and trustworthy resources. Now what? It's really important that you read through the stuff carefully and make notes as you go. This is for a number of reasons:

- You understand something a lot better if you write it down and have to explain it in your own words (when we argue it's the true test of understanding).

- It's easier to be organised and to find information when it comes to essays and revision.

- It will help you keep a record of your work and progress. You will know what you have read and what you thought about it.

- You can build up a record of accessible information – when you come to revise or use material in later years, you can't re-read every paper or every chapter in a book. Your notes will summarise the key issues in a few pages of writing.

- Even though it is that bit harder, in any kind of university work you do, it's always worth making sure you are engaging your brain. Reading through a paper can be a very passive activity – you might not really be paying attention, but can feel you are being productive. Taking notes as you go will make it active – it ensures you are thinking.

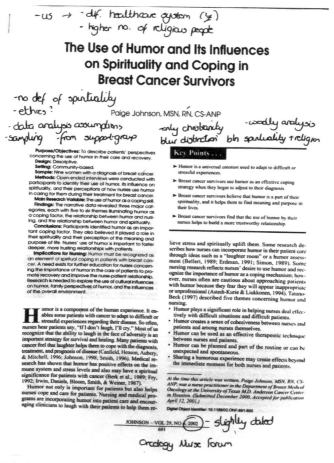

Figure 4.8 An example of effective notes and highlighting

A note on highlighting

When you're reading papers and journal articles, the temptation can be to print a copy and highlight relevant passages. However, often all you have done is turn the paper a different colour. It's important that you make some form of notes based on your reading – so summarise the information, draw out the key words and theories, and add your own thoughts. This will make it so much more meaningful to you when you come back to the paper.

Your own strategy for reading and note-taking

There are lots of reading and note-taking strategies. You might find these really useful and we wouldn't want to discourage you from investigating them. However, a word of caution: it's easy to get sidetracked by the technique as opposed to concentrating on the task in hand – you could spend longer reading about reading, or trying to apply the strategy, than going over the course material and making sense of it.

It's really important that you develop your *own* system for deciding what to read, doing the active reading, and making notes or highlights that will be of use in assessments and later years. You need something that is individual to you, that suits your learning preferences. As with note-taking in classes, there will be ways of working that play to your strengths. Do you like lists, shapes, colours? Do you prefer to highlight or copy out? Do you need everything to be in a hierarchical order or do you prefer a more scattered approach to information? Your system should incorporate those aspects of your personality.

BUT whatever your strategy, there are three things you really need to do:

1. **Always take a note of all the bibliographic details** (author, date, title, publisher, place of publication). Otherwise, you can't put the ideas or information into an assessment without going back and looking it all up again.

2. **Have a system for storing references**. For example, you could use a card file index where you note down details of the author, date,

title and publisher for each text consulted and put it in alphabetical order in a box on your desk. Ideally, add a little summary of what the text contains. There are also electronic systems, such as Refworks or Endnote. These can automatically upload or import references from your university's library catalogue or a database search. They can also complete a reference list for you to cut and paste on to the end of your essay. Details will be available on your university's library website.

3. **When making notes, put everything into your own words or use quotations.** Make clear where you have taken directly from a text, so that when you come to put things into the essay you know which are your own words and which you have to reference directly.

What to take from this chapter

- You can't say anything without evidence. That's why you search the literature, read it thoroughly and reference it within your assessments.

- Be careful what you read and include in your assessments. It's important to get a balance, but it has to be the right stuff. You are writing at university level, and all your assessments must be related to healthcare practice, so dodgy websites and questionable evidence are not appropriate and may even be dangerous.

- Printing out, photocopying or saving to your USB memory stick is not reading. You can feel you have tonnes of material and that you've done a good job, but unless you've read it and made meaningful notes it won't be any good to you.

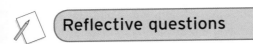

Reflective questions

1. List as many different sources of information as possible that you could potentially use when researching university work.

....

....

....

2. Are there sources you have relied on in the past that are no longer suitable? If so, why? Where will you turn instead?

....

....

....

3. Have a look at some past notes you have made (or quickly and roughly take notes on a newspaper article). What do they tell you about your learning preferences? Are they attractive and useful *for you* in the future? Can you adapt and develop your technique from them?

....

....

....

Further support

Your library will be your hub for information. Your librarian will be your friend (honestly, they don't bite!). Even if you don't physically sit in the building very often, you'll connect to eBooks and journals through their webpages. There will be loads of online tutorials and help pages as well as direct access to the resources. The library is also likely to offer drop-ins or face-to-face sessions to train you in finding resources.

The Internet Detective is a good online introduction to using the web for academic research.

http://www.vtstutorials.ac.uk/detective/

Feedback

Activity 4.1: Questioning the evidence

Here are our comments on the appropriateness of the news item for academic work:

1. The researchers claim that birds have a sense of humour, like that of humans.

2. An analysis of bird songs, after they have been shown 'humorous footage' of cats falling over.

3. Do we even know that birds can see video footage? How was the analysis conducted? How could they tell what the twittering represented? It may have been fear, confusion at being placed in front of a television? And who decided what defined 'humorous'?

4. Logically, we can't compare human psychological research with animal behaviour. They make huge claims about the entirety of the bird population based on a small research project.

5. We don't have any background to the research, or know about the qualifications of the researchers. Have the results been published in a peer-reviewed academic journal, as opposed to the popular press? And who, exactly, are the Avian Research Studies Executive?

6. The research is of questionable validity, and certainly wouldn't be suitable as evidence in academic work.

We think the most important thing for you to take away from this activity is that the news item is absolutely **not** suitable for university work. Perhaps the original piece of research is published in a peer-reviewed scholarly journal and may be of a suitable standard. But you would have to read it to find out.

Activity 4.2: Deciding on the suitability of sources

We would not consider any of these resources suitable for use as evidence in university work.

Wikipedia: It might be a good source for that quick fact check in a pub quiz or to settle a family argument, but it is not of appropriate quality for university work. We don't know who wrote the entry and therefore can't say much about whether they are qualified in this area. It can be easily changed, sometimes even maliciously. The problem is that you can't be sure enough of its accuracy to trust it.

NHS24: This is created by a reputable body and is held accountable for the information on it. But think of the intended audience. It is for patients to find out basic healthcare information. It is not for healthcare professionals. You hopefully expect to know more than your clients/ patients so you should be using more complex and detailed resources.

Mumsnet: Perhaps it's useful for parents but, again, where's the evidence base? Who is paying for this site (look at all of the adverts)? Are all inputs peer reviewed?

Nursing Standard* or *Nursing Times: These publications are written for the nursing community. They're like a newspaper containing reports on current affairs, rather than an academic journal. We recommend you read them, but they're not suitable for assessments.

Google: A good starting point for background knowledge, but it's no substitute for a database search. Ordering of the search returns is not neutral, but driven by popularity, advertising, etc., so you can be inadvertently influenced to look at the top hits. The same is true of Google scholar. So, by all means use it to find papers, but only as an additional search.

Chapter 5

Getting ready for academic writing

'I always thought of myself as a much more practical than academic person, so avoided writing. But once I was shown the rules, I was able to find my written voice.'

Second-year adult nursing student

LEARNING OUTCOMES

By the end of this chapter you should be able to:

- Describe the features of academic writing that distinguish it from other forms
- Apply the conventions of academic writing to your own work
- Justify why written communication is a lifelong learning skill for nursing

Introduction

This chapter will explain what makes academic writing ... well, academic writing: the rules you need to know about and obey, and advice for developing your writing style.

Academic writing conventions

Writing in university – both the stuff you'll read and the stuff you are expected to produce – is different from other kinds of writing in a number of ways. There are various rules and characteristics (conventions) of academic writing. In the same way that universitie are sometimes guilty of not explaining their language or assuming everyone knows what they are talking about, these rules of writing can often seem a bit hidden. You are expected to obey them, but no one may bother telling you what they are. So we will ...

ACTIVITY 5.1: DIFFERENT FORMS OF WRITING

Read through the following extracts. What makes the texts different from each other? Are there particular features?

Academic writing

> It is estimated that NHS annual expenditure on smoking-related diseases exceeds £4 billion (Department of Health 2011). Therefore, successive governments have invested in smoking cessation initiatives (World Health Organisation 2010). These have ranged from online support programmes (Smith 2008) to weekly group sessions in GP surgeries (Weston 2008).
>
> Whilst it is difficult to evaluate the impact of these programmes, as one factor among many in smokers' decisions to abstain (Lewis & Lee 2009), researchers have attempted to quantify success. Babbit and Dowser (2011) performed a longitudinal study on the impact of a smoking cessation programme in one NHS Trust. They reported that participants who had attended sessions were 10 per cent more likely to be living smoke free five

years later than those smokers who had registered an interest but failed to attend sessions. Though this may suggest that the programme brought health improvement benefits to the trust, Holmes and Goliath (2011) have argued that the results can be attributed to the stronger motivations of a self-selecting sample of participants – namely those who were committed enough to attend classes.

Journalistic writing

As revealed in the Herald and Star yesterday, cuts to the health budget have resulted in the closure of popular smoking cessation classes in GP surgeries. The 'Lung-Full' programme has been running for over three years, with hundreds of happy members who have kicked their habit since attending.

Lynsey Parker (35) is angry at yet more slashing of the local health budget and claims she would still be a smoker today without Lung-Full: 'My kids now live in a smoke-free home and I can climb the stairs without coughing,' she said. 'If these classes stop, who is going to help my wee sister quit?'

It has been proven that cessation classes make people twice as likely to stop smoking compared with nicotine patches or 'going cold turkey'. However, Councillor Tom Chalmers insists there simply isn't the money to fund these sorts of programmes.

Personal/blog writing

14 June – Just back from Docs about my back and had to walk past a bunch of scruffy protesters. So angry!!! They have the nerve to complain about closure of stop smoking classes!!! Why should my hard-earned tax money go to pay for their classes when all they need is a wee bit of gumption and a kick up the backside. I'm glad the funding's cut. Mebbe they can spend it on people with proper ailments now instead. I've not been able to work for years with this awful back of mine, but where's my classes!!!

See the feedback section at the end of the chapter for our thoughts on the extracts.

Features of academic writing

We think there are four main features of academic writing. If you understand and incorporate these into your own work, you'll develop a good academic tone.

The four features are:

1. Academic writing is clear and precise

Don't leave it up to your reader to make any conclusions. Be clear what you mean and state precisely what your argument is.

So, if you mean that A + B = C, don't just put in A and B and hope your reader works out that they = C.

State: A + B = C.

Other forms of writing can have multiple interpretations (five people may read a poem and all have a completely different understanding of it, which is what the poet may have wanted). However, academic writing should have no such vagueness. There should not be any reading between the lines.

Choose your words carefully so that the purpose and message is precise. *Report* means something slightly different from *allege*, *assert* or *insist*. The word you use depends on the strength of the comment you (or the researchers) are making.

2. Academic writing is objective/neutral/impersonal

Your work will be based on rational argument and evidence rather than your opinions or beliefs. You should try to remove yourself from the writing as much as possible and state things in a passive manner. This is very different from the forthright style of journalism or personal writing for example.

So avoid use of the first person (I, we, you, us). Instead of:

The report makes us think differently about how much what we eat affects diabetes ...

write:

> *The researchers suggest that, in fact, the link between diet and diabetes is not as clear as initially thought ...*

Instead of:

> *I looked through the literature and found that ...*

write

> *The literature search revealed that ...*

Most of the time you simply have to tweak what you're saying to make things more impersonal. It is about the evidence/information/theory rather than your take on it. This change in perspective can seem a bit strange, even artificial, but you soon get used to it.

3. Academic writing is formal

In order to improve clarity, etc., academic writing is very formal. There are a number of rules you simply have to obey.

- It is almost always written in prose (full sentences).
- You should never use abbreviations or contractions (instead of *couldn't, wouldn't, didn't,* write out *could not, would not, did not,* in full).
- Avoid slang (e.g. *dead good, total nightmare*). It's the difference between the way you would write a job application and the way you would speak to a friend.
- Watch out for colloquialisms or words that are very specific to your local area. Think about whether your writing is understandable to someone in another country or region. *The wean was in a dwaam (Glasgow). The l'aal babby had badly keppards (West Cumbria).* See what we mean!?
- Make sure you are not using judgemental language. For example, you wouldn't say that death rates were *appalling*. You may think so, but that's too informal and, ultimately, your opinion. Instead, you might say they were *significant* or *notable*.
- Spell out any acronyms or abbreviations the first time you use them within your text. So, for example, write Nursing and Midwifery

Council (NMC) in full at the start. Thereafter you can simply use NMC when referring to it. You are likely to use lots of acronyms and abbreviations in healthcare so make sure you provide a definition for the reader. They may not know who the WHO, RCN, HPC, NES and so on actually are.

If this all seems quite stressful and like a huge list to remember, don't worry. For the most part it's just about changing your language and vocabulary slightly.

ACTIVITY 5.2: FORMALISING YOUR VOCABULARY

What alternative words or expressions could you use to formalise your writing?

Instead of	Use
come up with	
look for	
sum up	
every year	
goes up	
goes down	
changes a lot	
put across	
think about	
look into	
on top of	

Turn to the feedback section at the end of this chapter to read our comments.

4. Academic writing provides evidence

As we've seen in previous chapters, it is essential that you provide evidence for everything you say at university. This is particularly true of written work. You will include references throughout to show where your information comes from and the evidence on which you are building your argument.

You can see from the examples of writing earlier in this chapter how different this makes academic writing. It is peppered with the names and publication dates of the authors whose work is used. At first, this can seem like it's interrupting the flow of the text, but it's absolutely vital. In comparison, the journalistic writing and blog examples make strong claims but do not provide any evidence to substantiate them. They also contain personal opinions and use more emotive language. You can see how this changes the overall tone or feel of the text.

Evidence and referencing

We've continually said that it's important to provide evidence to back up your arguments in academic work, and you do this by way of referencing. This is yet another academic convention that you'll have to get used to. As you write, you explicitly show the reader where you got your information from.

There are three reasons why you do this:

1. You need to use credible sources to show that your information is rigorous, and that you didn't just make it up. For example:

   Research suggests that in the 1980s British children drank sugary drinks on average once a week (Davies 2006). By 2005, this had increased to five times a week (Office of National Statistics 2007), which may partly explain the increased incidence in tooth decay (British Dental Association 2009).

2. To acknowledge the work of others. If you're putting together a playlist of songs, for example, you choose the order, the overall theme and whether you think the songs are good enough to go on it, but you'd never claim that you'd written or recorded the songs. If you don't say that it was Gibb's model of reflection, it's like you're saying you devised it. For example:

   Prensky's (2001) theory of Digital Immigrants has had a dramatic effect on educational theories and understanding the role of technology in learning.

3. To provide full bibliographic information to allow your reader to find the original material. They can then check accuracy and follow up any references. You follow one paper to another, to another

when researching. You are providing the same opportunity to your reader.

Referencing systems

There are several different referencing systems (that is, several different ways to reference in your writing). The one that you use will depend on your university, school or department, and possibly even the module. Make sure you find out how you are expected to reference before you start your first piece of work.

A couple of examples are given in Figures 5.1 and 5.2.

hence, presumably, an end: this had to be brought about by the action of those who were not interested in its eternity.[99]

Schlesinger believed that Marxism explained this situation and inspired and guided the movement that would remedy it. Marxism and its thinkers showed social-democracy how to organise to bring about revolution and how to construct a new state following that success. However, Marxism was also a philosophical methodology. Its historico-materialist outlook was a valid explanation of society and the way in which it operated. Marxism was a scientific method for scholarly pursuits, a way of understanding the world and investigating it. This method remained valid as circumstances changed and developed; Marxism was not a set of commandments or mere political

---

[96] Schlesinger, *Marxism-Leninism: An Outline* (Glasgow University Library, Rudolf Schlesinger Papers, MS Gen 1660, 49, Unpublished, 1968-1969). The preface detailed the origin of the book and the lectures (p. II).
[97] Schlesinger, *In a Time of Struggle: Whither Germany?*, p.93.
[98] Schlesinger, *Marxism-Leninism. Nine Lectures on Fundamentals*, (Glasgow University Library, Rudolf Schlesinger Papers, MS Gen 1660, 18, Unpublished, 1964-1966) 2, p. 1. Hereafter referred to as *Lectures*.
[99] Schlesinger, *Lectures*, 2, p. 2.

Figure 5.1 Vancouver numeric referencing system

The nature, and even existence, of CFS/ME has been an ongoing debate for decades (Wessely, Hotopf and Sharpe 1998; Working group on CFS/ME 2007). Much research regarding ME and those whom it affects acknowledges an origin that is post-viral (Deale, Chalder and Wessely 1998), and the role of physical attributions in treatment of the condition (Garralda and Range 2001; Deale, Chalder and Wessely 1998). Increasingly, however, interest has grown in the possibility of a psychogenic origin (Gordon 1988) and again, how this impacts on aetological attributions and the according effectiveness of treatment. However, whilst CFS/ME is now widely acknowledged as 'a real entity (which is) distressing, debilitating, and affects a very large number of people' (Calman 1998), a lack of physically obvious symptoms compromise recognition and identification of disabled people. Indeed, the unsympathetic 'yuppie flu' pseudonym attached to the condition from the late 1980s onwards demonstrates this widespread and very public skepticism.

Figure 5.2 Harvard bracketed referencing system

Regardless of the system you'll be using, there are always two parts to referencing:

1. The in-text reference/citation/footnote (the bit within the body of the text where you point out the source of information).

2. The reference list at the end (a complete list, arranged alphabetically by author's surname, of *all* the resources which have been cited in the text, with all of their bibliographical details (place of publication, full title, etc.).

People get really stressed about referencing. It's time consuming, pernickety and does take some getting used to. But just remember why you're doing it, and that will help with the technicalities. Could someone reading your work go and get hold of those sources themselves?

ACTIVITY 5.3: WHERE SHOULD THE REFERENCES GO?

We use references:

- to provide evidence to support ideas
- to credit the author
- to allow the reader to investigate further.

Where should the references go in the following text?

In the United Kingdom, it is calculated that between 30% and

40% of people who receive disability-related benefits would access further education if given the opportunity. Figures for Australia and Canada show similar results, 35% and 45% respectively.

Surveys suggest that charities consistently lobby government for greater funding to improve the educational options for this group. Yet, despite election promises, no policy on this matter has been published.

Turn to the feedback section at the end of this chapter to read our comment.

 Go to our companion website to try an online activity on finding the bibliographic details of a text.

A note on plagiarism

Plagiarism is taking someone else's work and passing it off as your own. This could involve buying an essay from the internet, copying large sections from a textbook, or taking bits of an essay from a student in the year above. This is clearly cheating, and as you'd expect, there would be consequences for the student involved.

However, sometimes it's possible to be accused of plagiarism because you haven't put things into your own words and shown where your evidence has come from. If you get to grips with referencing, and make sure you always acknowledge the source of your content, this shouldn't be a problem.

The Goldilocks approach to vocabulary and tone

It's important that you get the balance *juuuust right* in the breadth of vocabulary you use. You shouldn't use too simplistic language, but equally it shouldn't read like you swallowed a thesaurus. It needs to be of sufficient variety to demonstrate knowledge and be interesting to the reader. However, it does need to be YOUR words and YOUR understanding of a topic, so don't put in terminology and concepts that you don't understand.

ACTIVITY 5.4: GETTING THE BALANCE

Read the following examples to see what we mean:

Example 1

What do u have to no to right an essay for university? I'd start by righting everything I no about a subject then putting it in a list then making some headings to divide up the information into wee bits. And I'd get books on the list that chris gave me so I'd no what background information to put in cause that'd help people see the bigger picture and make them think about how it relates to the essay which I wouldn't have chose myself cause it was dead boring.

Comments on Example 1:

....

....

....

Example 2

Specific semantic conventions exist within the overarching structure of composition within the Higher Education sector as regards the production of text-based assessment. Interrogation and consultation of a systematic, yet not exhaustive, list of resources; possibly texts themselves, or presented in an alternate, multimodal manifestation, will suitably ensure that those engaged in a dedicated educational endeavour espouse with eloquence within the negotiated parameters of the subject area.

Comments on Example 2:

....

....

....

Example 3

Academic writing is a term used for different types of written assessments in university (James 2010). Though there are many different types of academic writing (Entwistle 2008), such as an essay, there are certain conventions which are consistent throughout. These include keeping sentences short and to the point, as well as avoiding jargon and colloquialisms. It is also important that students refer to the reading list given to them at the beginning of a module. This will ensure that key information within the subject area is incorporated and that the piece of writing is put in context (Banks 2007).

Comments on Example 3:

....

....

....

We've provided our own comments in the feedback section, but it's hopefully pretty clear that Example 3 is the most balanced and appropriate for university work.

A note on grammar

Good writing isn't about trying to sound clever. It's about getting your meaning across in as straightforward a way as you can. Often shorter sentences are best. Do you really need five words when one could be just as effective?

It's the same with grammar. We're not saying you need to be the world's best user of an apostrophe, but be aware of sentence structure and how punctuation can change meaning. Know what your weaknesses are and spend time proof-reading. Maybe you know that you just can't help adding commas everywhere, in which case, when reading through your work, check every comma. The chances are that many could be replaced with a full stop or simply removed. Reading aloud is always a good idea to check the clarity of your writing.

Common mistakes in academic writing

1. Long sentences

Students can fall into the trap of simply putting in commas rather than finishing sentences. Often it seems to come from a lack of confidence, but it can make your writing difficult to understand. For example:

> *Healthcare professionals work collaboratively in a variety of settings, including hospital wards and many different areas of the community (Henderson 2001), and do so as part of a large, multidisciplinary team, who have a variety of expertise and subject-specific knowledge to help them provide the best care possible to patients in each clinical area.*

The text reads easier when punctuated:

> *Healthcare professionals work collaboratively in a variety of settings, including hospital wards and many different areas of the community (Henderson 2001). They do so as part of a large, multidisciplinary team. Team members have a variety of expertise and subject-specific knowledge to help them provide the best care possible to patients in each clinical area.*

2. Unlinked concepts

Your writing should be a logical discussion and your reader should be able to see why you're including each point. Students can sometimes state a point and then another, but fail to show how they are related (so, again, if you mean A + B = C, say it). For example:

> *In order to provide the best possible patient care, written and oral communication skills are vital (Floyd 2002). Florence Nightingale was a pioneer of her time for the advances she promoted in improved hygiene and ventilation.*

These two sentences seem to be on completely unrelated topics. The author may well have a link in their mind, but they need to make it obvious.

3. Mistakes that your spellchecker won't notice

For example, *their, there, they're; to, too, two.* Spellcheckers are really useful, but are not without their flaws. They don't know what you intended to write, and often won't pick up different versions of words in the wrong context. It's important that you re-read your work to ensure it's as accurate as it can be. For example:

> *One of the first assessment tasks for clinical staff is to take personal information form the patient being admitted.*

Here, *form* is not an incorrectly spelled word, so your spellchecker may not pick it up. It should, of course, be *from*.

4. Incomplete sentences

What we mean by this is that there's no subject, object and verb. We don't want to give you an English language lesson, but by reading your work aloud, you'll be able to tell when a sentence is a sentence, or if something is missing. For example:

> *In order to gain consent and ensure legal obligations are met, as well as obeying the code of conduct.*

This is not a sentence. *In order to gain consent*, then what? How about:

> *In order to gain consent and ensure legal obligations are met, as well as obeying the code of conduct, the receiving nurse should verify signatures on treatment forms.*

> ## Why do I have to spend so much time developing my writing?

We know that you are joining your degree to become a nurse rather than a student, but it's really important that you can write clearly. Not just at university, but throughout your career. Think about all the times you'll be required to write:

● patient notes, shift handovers and team communication

- reports and recommendations for practice
- job applications.

Each of these types of writing will have different readers, but you still need to make a convincing, detailed and logical argument.

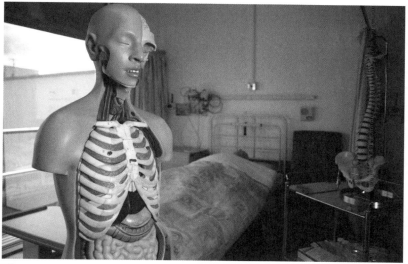

Figure 5.3 The clinical area
(Source: Angus Forbes, copyright Glasgow Caledonian University)

ACTIVITY 5.5: CASE NOTES

Read through these three examples of case notes:

Case notes: example 1	Case notes: example 2	Case notes: example 3
11 April, 9 am	11 April, 9 am	11 April, 9 am
Slept alright but a wee bit of tossing and turning. No drink.	Slept well through the night, at least six hours, although did have to visit the bathroom twice. Offered water to drink at 7 am but declined.	Despite two visits to the bathroom, the patient slept well for two four-hour intervals and claims to feel much more relaxed as a result. Declined fluids at 7 am in order to continue sleeping but has requested tea and dry toast.

Figure 5.4 Case note examples

Which of the examples conveys the most detailed and accurate information? Does this matter? Are there implications for the care of the patient? What kind of case notes do you hope to write in professional practice?

Turn to the feedback section at the end of this chapter to read our comments.

It might feel as if there's a lot of work in developing your writing, and essays may seem very artificial and a long way from nursing practice, but the skills themselves are important.

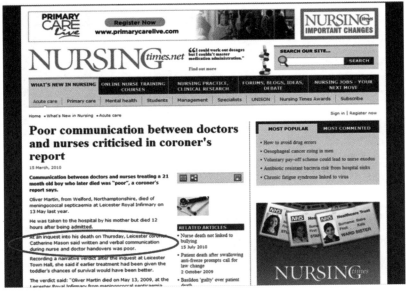

Figure 5.5 Media report on poor communication

(Source: www.nursingtimes.net, Nursing Times)

The example in Figure 5.5 shows one of the consequences a breakdown in communication might have on patient care.

As you can see from the job advert in Figure 5.6, you need writing skills as well as all your clinical competencies once you graduate. In fact, you need those skills to complete the application form effectively and to even get your foot in the door.

Candidate information

> Ref no: L/440/72
>
> Post: Community Addictions Psychiatric Staff Nurse
>
> Location: Multiple
>
> Closing date for applications: 31st May

This post is for a fixed term of 6 months.

Hours of work (37.5 per week) will be negotiated with the successful candidate.

Knowledge, experience and required qualifications

> - You must be a registered nurse in mental health, with proof of a valid registration with the Nursing and Midwifery Council.
> - You will be required to demonstrate a sound understanding of addiction related theory.
> - You must be able to provide evidence of your commitment to continuing professional development.
> - Experience of working in the field of addictions or in a community setting is essential.
> - *You will have excellent communication skills.*
> - IT skills are essential.
> - You will hold a full current driving licence.

Figure 5.6 Importance of written communication from an employer's perspective

What to take from this chapter

- Don't try too hard to sound clever. You'll demonstrate your intelligence through clear writing on complex topics.

- Make sure there's a purpose to every sentence you write. Is it clear to the reader?

- Consider the formal style other authors use. If you're finding a textbook or journal paper particularly difficult or easy to understand, why is that? Is it something to do with the writing style?

- Read a broadsheet rather than a tabloid. It could widen your vocabulary and introduce you to a formal style of writing.

- Make sure you show where all your evidence comes from, and apply the referencing system that your university uses.

Reflective questions

1. List the features of academic writing.

....

....

....

2. Consider your own writing. Are there mistakes you always make, or things that you know you're good at in academic writing (for example, how's your punctuation)? Are there any areas you need to focus on?

....

....

....

3. In what ways will improving your writing now help you be a better nurse in the future?

....

....

....

Further support

Your university will provide support for academic writing in some form or other. It may be a centralised writing unit or staff located within your school or department who specialise in working with students to improve their writing. Have a look on your institution's website to see what's available. Even if you don't want to see someone in person, there are often handouts and web pages, or you could always email for a bit of advice.

There are also lots of study guides available:

Cowen, M., Maier, P. and Price, G. (2009). *Study Skills for Nursing and Healthcare Students*, Pearson Education Ltd.

Feedback

Activity 5.1: Different forms of writing

A quick read through the texts should show you just how different types of writing can be. Among other things, their tone, vocabulary, structure and formality all vary.

Activity 5.2: Formalising your vocabulary

Here are some suggestions for formalising informal language. Please note this is not an exhaustive list; there are lots of other possibilities that you could use. These are just some ideas to get you thinking.

Instead of	Use
come up with	develop, devise, establish, suggest, produce
look for	investigate, research, consider
sum up	conclude, summarise
every year	annually, per annum
goes up	increases
goes down	decreases
changes a lot	varies, fluctuates
put across	convey, communicate
think about	consider, analyse, evaluate
look into	research, investigate, examine
on top of	additionally, in addition, furthermore

Activity 5.3: Where should the references go?

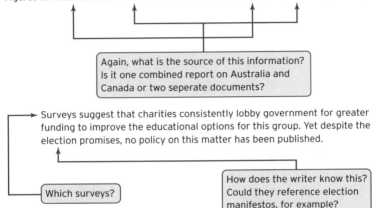

> This is a very precise figure – where is the evidence? We would expect to see a reference showing the source of the information.

In the United Kingdom, it is calculated that between 30% and 40% of people who receive disability-related benefits would access further education if given the opportunity. Figures for Australia and Canada show similar results, 35% and 45% respectively.

> Again, what is the source of this information? Is it one combined report on Australia and Canada or two seperate documents?

Surveys suggest that charities consistently lobby government for greater funding to improve the educational options for this group. Yet despite the election promises, no policy on this matter has been published.

> Which surveys?

> How does the writer know this? Could they reference election manifestos, for example?

Figure 5.7 Where do the references go? – some suggestions

Activity 5.4: Getting the balance

Comments on Example 1:

This is not written in English, never mind academic English:

- there is use of the first person (lots of 'I')
- there are spelling mistakes (it should be *know* not *no*)
- it uses both judgemental and informal language (*dead boring*)
- there are no references to substantiate any arguments (who is Chris, for example?).

Comments on Example 2:

This piece of writing seems so busy trying to sound clever that it loses any meaning:

- it uses as many words as possible when one precise one might have been better (rather than *interrogation and consultation*, how about *use of*?)
- as with the first text, there are no references. Where is the evidence for what is being said?

Comments on Example 3:
This is a balanced piece of academic writing:

- the tone is formal but the meaning is very clear and simple
- there is good use of evidence
- the purpose of each statement is precise and relevant.

Activity 5.5: Case notes

We hope you agree that the third example provides a lot more detail regarding the patient. The more information you have, and the more effective the communication, the better the patient care.

Chapter 6

Getting ready for the essay writing process

'It was great when I realised that pretty much every essay at university has the same structure. You just need to think about the reader all the time.'

Third-year adult nursing student

LEARNING OUTCOMES

By the end of this chapter you should be able to:

- Use an essay writing process to help you tackle your first assessment
- Plan and structure your written work
- Develop your own proof-reading checklist for use with your assessments

Introduction

In this chapter we recommend breaking the assessment process down into several stages. We argue that the structure of your written work is as important as the content.

The essay writing process

Whether you are working on an essay, a case study or a presentation, there is a clear process to producing the assessment.
The four stages of that process are:

1. Analyse the question or task – spend time working out exactly what is being asked of you.

2. Get the content and plan – search the literature, gather resources and think about how you will build your argument.

3. Put it together – do the writing, possibly with several drafts.

4. Edit – proof-read the work to check whether it answers the question, makes sense, etc.

Using a process like this has several advantages:

- Things are broken into smaller, more manageable pieces. This can help with motivation or getting you started if it all feels too big to handle.

- Time management becomes easier. You can allot time for each stage of the process and keep an eye on whether you are falling behind.

- Your work should become more structured and polished because you've spent time planning and editing. These things are easily missed out if you hurtle headlong into the assessment.

- It is the same process whatever the assessment. So the more you use it, the better you will be at completing work on time and in a structured, stress-free way.

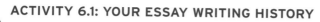

ACTIVITY 6.1: YOUR ESSAY WRITING HISTORY

Think about an assessment you completed successfully in the past.

1. What were the different tasks involved? How did you get from knowing the work was due to having the assessment written and ready to submit? For example, did you have to go and find resources? Did you write a plan?

....

....

....

....

2. Were you aware of the different stages of that process? Did you break the overall task down into smaller bits?

....

....

....

....

3. If you were to go through the process again would you do anything differently?

....

....

....

....

Turn to the feedback section at the end of this chapter to read our comments.

In our experience (and we read an awful lot of essays), we can always tell when someone has followed a writing process, spent time unpicking the question, thought about a plan and left time for redrafting. These essays are always better structured and easier to read.

Go to our companion website to view an example of planning for written assessments. We've also provided a blank template for you to use when you have your own assessment to plan.

Writing an essay: what to know, ask and do

1. Analyse the question

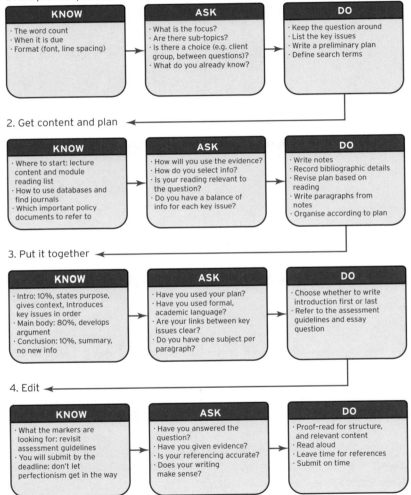

KNOW	ASK	DO
· The word count · When it is due · Format (font, line spacing)	· What is the focus? · Are there sub-topics? · Is there a choice (e.g. client group, between questions)? · What do you already know?	· Keep the question around · List the key issues · Write a preliminary plan · Define search terms

2. Get content and plan

KNOW	ASK	DO
· Where to start: lecture content and module reading list · How to use databases and find journals · Which important policy documents to refer to	· How will you use the evidence? · How do you select info? · Is your reading relevant to the question? · Do you have a balance of info for each key issue?	· Write notes · Record bibliographic details · Revise plan based on reading · Write paragraphs from notes · Organise according to plan

3. Put it together

KNOW	ASK	DO
· Intro: 10%, states purpose, gives context, Introduces key issues in order · Main body: 80%, develops argument · Conclusion: 10%, summary, no new info	· Have you used your plan? · Have you used formal, academic language? · Are your links between key issues clear? · Do you have one subject per paragraph?	· Choose whether to write introduction first or last · Refer to the assessment guidelines and essay question

4. Edit

KNOW	ASK	DO
· What the markers are looking for: revisit assessment guidelines · You will submit by the deadline; don't let perfectionism get in the way	· Have you answered the question? · Have you given evidence? · Is your referencing accurate? · Does your writing make sense?	· Proof-read for structure, and relevant content · Read aloud · Leave time for references · Submit on time

Figure 6.1 The essay writing process

Stage one: analyse the question

It may sound odd, but it's a good idea to really spend time unpicking the assessment task. It is just so easy to misremember the question, only answer half of it, or spend ages writing about the topic you hoped was set rather than the one that actually was.

Sometimes you will be given a very specific essay question. Sometimes you may actually choose the focus yourself. For others, you may be asked to discuss a particular clinical scenario or case study. Whatever the precise nature of the task, you will be given information about the topic and what is expected of you (often called the assessment guidelines). Pay attention to these and keep them around you.

What is the overall topic you are investigating? And what are the specifics? Do you have to choose a particular field of nursing (e.g. child, mental health, etc.) or client group, for example?

Having decided that, begin to ask yourself a series of questions – brainstorm the issue:

- Do you need to define any terms? Are there any contentious issues?
- What is the overall context of the question? Why have you been asked to cover this subject?
- What theories underpin any discussion of the topic?
- What themes come to mind? From reading/lectures, etc?
- Have you had any relevant placement experiences?
- Where will you search for resources? What search terms? What selection/inclusion criteria? How up to date? Which countries? Which journals?

The reason you do all this is so that, eventually, you produce a well thought-out, structured essay that answers all aspects of the question and stays on topic.

For example, you have been given the following essay question/task:

Discuss the extent to which nurses can play a key role in the prevention of hospital-acquired infections (HAIs).

If you spend time analysing the question, you'll see it consists of three parts:

(a) Hospital acquired infections

(b) The *prevention* of hospital acquired infections

(c) The role of the nurse (in b).

All three of these areas have to be addressed if you are to pass the assessment. It's also vital that you get the balance between the different topics. This essay is likely to talk broadly about what HAIs are, but you must focus on prevention (rather than treatment, for example). You also have to pay enough attention to what this means for nursing- how can *the nurse* prevent HAIs?

A quick glance at the question, and a desire to get on with things, might have sent you researching HAIs. If your essay only discussed that topic, however good it was, it would not have met all the assessment criteria (and you wouldn't get a good mark).

A note on marking/assessment criteria

As well as looking at the assessment guidelines in this first stage of the process, you should think about who will be reading your work. You are not writing for the sake of it; you are writing so that your knowledge and understanding can be assessed (marked/judged/evaluated). So it makes good sense to be aware of what the markers are looking for.

Ideally, you will be given this information by your module tutor. You may even be given the marking grid or guidelines that they will use to mark the assessments. This would typically tell you how the marks are broken down (how many for structure, how many for content, for example).

The more you know about what the markers would like from you, the more you can ensure you give them exactly that. Don't be afraid to ask how your work will be assessed. Marking shouldn't be some big secret and tutors will be happy to discuss this with you.

Again, keep this information close to hand. Keep returning to the assessment guidelines and the marking criteria throughout the writing process. You can then check you're still on the right track.

Stage two: get content and plan

Having figured out what is being asked of you and your initial thoughts and knowledge on the subject, the next stage of essay writing involves gathering information. We've already discussed searching the literature and the importance of finding appropriate evidence in Chapter 4.

But after that stage ... STOP!!!

Most people have a tendency to rush straight into writing once they've found the content. Some even start writing while they are doing their reading. This isn't to be recommended. At this point you really need to spend time gathering your thoughts, thinking about what the key themes are, how they fit together, what order you should discuss things in and how your essay should look. Basically, you need to develop a plan.

Plans ensure:

- you answer the question
- you don't just randomly jump from one sub-topic to another
- you provide a conclusion for your points
- you include sufficient evidence.

Plans give your work structure and a logical order that's clear for a reader to follow. They are also really great for breaking down the task so that none of it is intimidating. Suddenly you aren't faced with a blank screen and 1500 words to write. You have a list of sub-topics and know that you only need to write perhaps 300 words for each – much less scary!

You can plan in lots of different ways. Find a method that suits your learning. You may wish to devise a mindmap so you can see all of the themes and how they interrelate. Others may prefer to write a bulleted list of paragraph topics. In our view, the more detailed the plan the better. You might want a plan that lists the theme of each paragraph, the sub-topics, what evidence you will include and how you will relate everything back to the role of the nurse and the overall essay question.

Planning the essay: tools

These diagrams show a few different ways to plan assessments. The example looks at a 1500-word essay on reflective practice.

- Introduction
- Define reflective theory
- Why reflection important in healthcare
- Overview of three main models
- Gibbs
- Johns
- Rolfe *et al.*
- Compare and contrast
- Conclusion

Figure 6.2 A bulleted list

Introduction
- *State the aim of the essay*
- *Outline what the essay will cover and in what order*

Paragraph 2: define reflective theory
- *What is reflective theory?*
- *How does it relate to healthcare?*
- *What is a reflective practitioner?*

Paragraph 3: overview of three main models
- *Introduce Gibbs, Johns and Rolfe et al.*

Paragraph 4: Gibbs
- *Gibbs' model in detail*
- *Main features: stages, dynamic cycle*
- *Developed in education*

Paragraph 5: Johns
- *Johns' model in detail*
- *Main features: looking in and looking out*
- *Developed in practice*

Paragraph 6: Rolfe
- *Rolfe et al. model in detail*
- *Main feature: three key questions*
- *Which is most key?*

Paragraph 7: compare and contrast
- *What are the commonalities/ differences between models?*
- *How does this affect validity/use?*

Conclusion
- *Sum up*
- *Link back to question*

Figure 6.3 An expanded paragraph plan

Page 1	Page 2
Introduction (approx. 150 words): • *State the aim of the essay* • *Outline what the essay will cover and in what order* Paragraph 2: the development of reflective theory (approx. 200 words) • *Where and when were concepts of reflection developed?* • *Who are the main theorists?*	Paragraph 3: reflection as a dynamic process (approx. 200 words) • *Cycles as a main feature* • *ERA at macro-structure* Paragraph 4: reflection in professionalism (approx. 200 words) • *Examples* • *Gibbs: developed in education* • *Johns: developed in clinical area*
Page 3	**Page 4**
Paragraph 5: reflection-in-action vs reflection-on-action (approx. 200 words) • *Schon 1983* • *How does stage affect reflection?* • *Development of 'same time' reflective skills* Paragraph 6: Applying reflective models in practice (approx. 200 words) • *Reflection in the clinical scenario* • *Enablers/inhibitors* • *The importance of action plans*	Paragraph 7: Tools for reflection (approx. 200 words) • *Systematic observations* • *Diaries, professional development activities* • *Sharing reflective experiences* Conclusion (approx. 150 words) • *Sum up* • *Link back to question* • *Demonstrate learning*

Figure 6.4 A word count plan

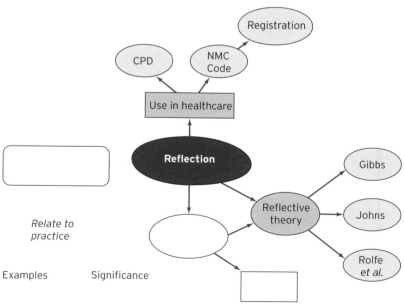

Figure 6.5 A mindmap plan

Stage three: put it together

Every piece of written academic work is made up of the same components. There's an introduction, main body, conclusion, and references.

Introduction: As you might have guessed, this is where you introduce the piece of work. You re-state the question, explain how you're going to answer it and give an overview of sub-topics in the order they will be covered. If you have had to make any choices in answering the question (for example, care of a particular patient group) you will detail this. You may also provide a rationale or justification to support your decisions. Typically the introduction will be about 10–15 per cent of your essay (so, in a 1500-word essay, around 150–200 words).

Main body: This is the meat of the writing. It's where you present your case and outline and discuss the main themes. You'll divide the main body into paragraphs, making sure that you have shown how the topics interrelate and, indeed, are relevant to the overall question.

A note on paragraphs

People can get very stressed by paragraphs – we're always being asked how long they should be, and some people fail to use them altogether. But it's pretty straightforward, really. It's dividing your ideas into manageable sub-topics, allowing the reader to understand when there's a change in subject, and also giving their eyes a rest by breaking the text up.

Each paragraph should have a clear topic sentence that introduces the subject. If you're moving on to a new topic, or a new aspect of the original one, think about starting a new paragraph. There's not really any ideal length, but it must be more than one sentence, and you would expect to have at least a couple to each word-processed page of A4.

Conclusion: This is where you'll summarise your discussion and the key points you want the reader to take away. It's often worth re-stating the question, and showing how you have answered or addressed it. This section will not include any new information. Sometimes people are misled by the word 'conclusion' – any conclusion, recommendations or implications should come towards the end of the main body, once you've presented your evidence. Again, typically, the conclusion will comprise of 10-15 per cent of your overall word count. So:

Say what you're going to say (introduction).

Say it (main body).

Say it again (conclusion).

References/reference list: The vast majority of assessments also require a full list of all of the resources (books, journal articles, etc.) you have used and referred to within it. This is typically at the end of the essay, and ordered alphabetically by author's surname.

Remember: As much as we're saying you, you, you – don't forget, you rarely, if ever, use the first person in academic writing, so you won't be saying 'I'.

Why bother with a structure?

Planning and sticking to these components of academic work is important. They're just as much an academic convention as making sure your writing is formal and objective.

In your written work, you're building an argument. You should be leading your reader through this, pretty much by the hand. You show them how the topics are linked, demonstrating their implications explicitly by having a logical structure and providing signposts. You need to make sure your reader doesn't get lost halfway through.

The other reason you need a structure is because there's so much information to include. You need to order it somehow, and make that visible to the reader.

When structuring the main body, it's useful to think about moving from the big to the small. Initially, you need to provide context and set the scene. It's also worth a discussion of why the topic is important – not for you personally, but from an academic and professional rationale.

You then move on to your main points, the big themes and issues in the field. You should provide evidence and include examples to give further detail and introduce discussion.

And so on, through to the lesser topics.

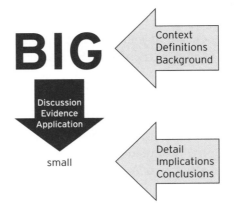

Figure 6.6 From the big to the small

A note on the order of your topics

Remember, you are not writing a murder mystery! Students often make the mistake of leaving their best arguments, the main points, to the very end. There isn't a big reveal of the killer – at no stage should your reader be surprised by what's coming. This is another thing that can feel strange as you develop your writing style, but it's yet one more convention. It's about having clarity in your work, and explicitly stating your point.

When you haven't planned or thought about structure, the reader can be left confused. Essays can jump from one topic to another, seemingly at random. There can be lots of repetition (and that's really wasteful when you have a limited word count) and vital parts of the question can be left unaddressed. Figure 6.7 shows, on the left, an essay which has a clear plan and structure. The essay on the right does not.

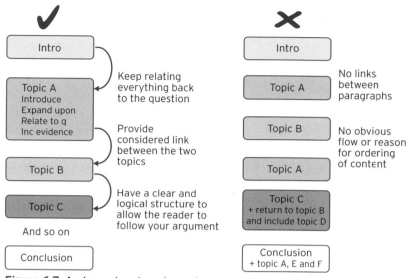

Figure 6.7 A planned and unplanned essay

ACTIVITY 6.2: AN EXAMPLE ESSAY

To what extent do reflective models improve the practice of healthcare professionals?

The following essay contains relevant content and is written in a formal, academic tone. However, it is difficult to follow because it lacks structure. It could be improved simply by reordering the information so that topics are dealt with in a logical and clear way.

Go through the essay and note down the topics covered. Then suggest how the sentences and paragraphs could be rearranged to improve structure.

Main points:

1 Intro – definition of reflection and description of what essay will cover.

2 Reflective practice – broad definitions

3 ....

4 ....

5 ....

6 ....

```
..........................................
..........................................
..........................................
..........................................
..........................................
..........................................
..........................................
..........................................
..........................................
..........................................
```

Reflection is the process of internally examining and exploring an issue (Boyd & Fales 1983). It involves consciously considering experiences, actions and feelings and then interpreting them to facilitate learning in the future (Boud et al. 1994). This essay will explore the principles of reflection and consider the importance of the concept for healthcare professionals, with particular reference to nurses.

It will consider a number of reflective models and discuss the ways in which they aid nurses in becoming reflective practitioners before examining evidence to suggest that models may, in fact, inhibit the development of reflective skills. Reflective practice is a complex concept that has been defined in many ways (Rogers 2009, Reid 2001, Lloyd 1999).

```
..........................................
..........................................
..........................................
..........................................
..........................................
..........................................
..........................................
..........................................
..........................................
```

Reflective practice is considered one of the cornerstones of modern nursing (Gillies 2007). For Jacques (2005), in an ever-changing social and healthcare environment, the ability of nurses to continually improve and update their practice is vital, and is enshrined in profes-sional codes and standards (Nursing Midwifery Council (NMC 2006, NMC 2007)).

At its core, it involves practitioners learning from their experiences through the considered exploration and analysis of those events in order to inform their practice in the future.

```
.............................
.............................
.............................
.............................
.............................
.............................
.............................
.............................
.............................
.............................
```

For Beattie, it is 'the mirror through which nurses can focus on themselves in a constructive, developmental manner. It allows professionals to integrate theory and reality, and work towards an ideal model of practice' (2000, p. 34).

Reflection is considered one of the best tools for the improvement of practice (Livingstone 2004). In addition, Lee et al. (2010) argue that if nursing is to become the professionalised occupation an all-degree status can afford it, it is essential practitioners engage in continuous and recordable professional development. Again, they argue that this is best achieved through reflective practice.

```
.............................
.............................
.............................
.............................
.............................
.............................
.............................
.............................
.............................
.............................
```

A number of models exist to guide practitioners through the stages of the reflective process in a structured way (Michaels 2006). Perhaps the most commonly used within nursing (Evans & Betts 2009) is Gibbs' (1988) reflective cycle. As the name implies, this is a circular model that asks a series of questions about the incident, the practitioner's feelings, their analysis and, ultimately, their learning plans for the future. According to Lewis et al. (2003) one of its main strengths is that it promotes action planning in this way. Johns' (2000) model of structured reflection and Rolfe's (2001) framework for reflective practice are also frequently utilised by nurses (Michaels 2006).

```
.....................................
.....................................
.....................................
.....................................
.....................................
.....................................
.....................................
.....................................
.....................................
.....................................
```

Reflective models appear to improve the practice of nurses in a number of ways. Reflection can be a difficult skill to acquire and, according to Newark and Marine (2010), novice nurses in particular can find it difficult at first. Models provide structure and guidance as practitioners begin reflection. North London NHS Trust (2009), for example, recommends that newly qualified student nurses develop their practice with use of Gibbs' model. They argue the guidance offered in this step-by-step approach, 'helps nurses see the links between theory and practice, your feelings and actions' (2009, p. 45).

```
.....................................
.....................................
.....................................
.....................................
.....................................
.....................................
.....................................
.....................................
.....................................
.....................................
```

Whilst there is a large body of evidence to suggest that reflective models improve practice, some argue that their use can have a negative impact on healthcare professionals. Lurey and Wilder (2007) call for less rigid teaching of reflection within nursing education. They argue that current models inhibit personal learning styles and often lead to mechanistic, 'box ticking' exercises rather than a genuine consideration of the nursing role. Similarly, Tupay (2003) asserts that reflective models are overused in nursing.

```
..................................
..................................
..................................
..................................
..................................
..................................
..................................
..................................
..................................
..................................
..................................
```

Models are also often used to ensure that learning takes place through reflection, and so practice improves. Trout et al. (2007) argue that practitioners all too easily mistake reflection for 'indulgent navel gazing', concentrating on their feelings rather than analysing events, searching for meaning and learning for the future. Models structure reflection so that analysis and action planning are distinct phases in the process. Their use maintains the positive, learning elements of the activity (Barros 2001).

In conclusion ...

Turn to the feedback section to see how we think the essay should have been structured. Does it make it easier to read and follow? Do you think it would have received a higher mark? We do. The content of the two essays is exactly the same. The only difference is the order in which the information is written. This shows just how important it is to plan, structure and provide signposts for your reader.

Several ways to skin a cat

Two different students working on the same assessment will find very different resources and, therefore, develop different plans and different structures. So don't panic if, in talking to your friends, their essays seem nothing like yours. You may all be on the right track – and there's no reason to think that you're the one who's got it wrong.

The important things are that:

- you've searched the literature and evaluated your resources critically
- you've analysed the question and spent time planning
- you've provided a clear rationale where appropriate
- there's a logical structure to your work.

Have a read through the two essay plans below. They are fairly different from each other but both demonstrate a thorough interpretation of the question and a reasoned structure.

'Discuss the extent to which nurses can play a key role in the prevention of hospital acquired infections'

Introduction
- Outline purpose of essay and how it will be structured

Section 1 (background):
- Definition of HAIs
- Healthcare context
- Implications for healthcare – impact on patients, costs etc.

Section 2:
- Nurse's role in preventing spread of HAIs through care given
- Examples in practice

Section 3:
- Nurse's role in preventing spread through education
- Examples in practice

Section 4:
- Discussion of who else in team plays a key role and limitations to the nurse's role in this respect
- Implications, recommendations

Conclusion:
- Summarise key points and finish by stating to what extent the statement in the question is true

---

Figure 6.8 Possible structure 1

> **Introduction:**
> - Outline purpose of essay and how it will be structured
>
> **Section 1 (background):**
> - Definition of HAIs
> - Healthcare context
> - Implications for healthcare – impact on patients, costs etc.
>
> **Section 2:**
> - Presentation of evidence showing nurses do play key role
> - Discussion of why this is the case
> - Examples of this in practice, e.g. hand-washing policies, use of protective equipment
>
> **Section 3:**
> - Presentation of evidence showing limitations to nurse's role in preventing HAIs
> - Discussion of why this is the case and what the drawbacks/ problems in practice may be
>
> **Section 4:**
> - Summarise arguments for and against the nurse's role being the key factor
>
> **Conclusion:**
> - Summarise key points and finish by stating to what extent the statement in the question is true

Figure 6.9 Possible structure 2

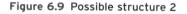

Stage four: edit

The final stage in the writing process involves the proof-reading of your work. This is a really important part of the essay writing process, and can easily be overlooked or avoided. Having spent so much time building and writing your argument, the last thing you may want to do is go over your essay with a critical eye. However, it is well worth investing a few hours at this point to make sure that your essay is the best it can be.

Where possible, finish writing a couple of days before the deadline so you can give yourself a bit of time away from the essay before coming back with a fresh perspective.

The following checklist should help you think about all of the areas you need to cover.

Structure	Yes	No	Action?
Do I have an introduction, main body and conclusion?			
Does my introduction give an overview of the essay?			
Is there a logical flow to my argument in the main body?			
Do I have one sub-topic per paragraph?			
Are the links between sub-topics clear?			
Does my conclusion summarise the key points?			
Content	Yes	No	Action?
Have I followed the assessment guidelines?			
Have I answered the question?			
Have I demonstrated wide reading through references?			
Are most references less than five years old?			
Have I included evidence for each definition/statement?			
Are my in-text references accurate?			
Have I considered implications for nursing?			
Style	Yes	No	Action?
Is my writing in a clear, formal and academic tone?			
Have I avoided using 'I' or 'we'?			
Have I written out acronyms in full on their first use?			
Have I taken care over grammar and punctuation?			
Is my writing in sentences?			
Are paragraphs an appropriate length?			
Format	Yes	No	Action?
Have I used the appropriate font and line spacing?			
Have I ensured I am within the word count?			
Is my reference list accurate and complete?			
Have I used a spell-checker?			
Am I ready to submit by the deadline?			
Do I know whether to submit a paper or electronic copy?			

Figure 6.10 Proof-reading checklist

Proof-reading dos and don'ts

 Try to give yourself at least an evening away from your work so that you can come back to it with fresh eyes.

Use or develop a proof-reading checklist.

Get to know your common errors and look out for these.

Know what spellcheckers won't pick up (*there, their, they're*).

Don't become a perfectionist and keep reading your essay over and over.

Don't run out of steam at this final stage. Effective proof-reading makes the difference between a poor or satisfactory essay and a really good one.

Whilst it can be helpful to have someone else read your work over, ultimately the decision as to whether it's ready to hand in has to be yours.

ACTIVITY 6.3: CARELESS WRITING

As we've seen, proof-reading is an important part of the essay writing process and can be easily overlooked. By leaving a bit of time before submission you can correct mistakes that are easy to make when the pressure is on. Grammatical errors, typos and careless punctuation can all compromise the first impression your marker has of your work. Lack of attention to detail can also result in your changing the meaning of what you're writing, which could have serious implications for practice. It's worth making the effort so that your writing is as accurate as it can be.

Comment on the following aspects of the extract:

Spelling: ....

Grammar and punctuation: ....

Clarity of writing style: ....

Formality of writing style: ....

There are threee important aspects to clinical decision making requires three things. Firstly, practitioners should have an up date knowledge or practice int their area expertise (Smith 2008). We can then be sure that they have all the information they need to deliver appropriate care to a specific client group Secondly clear and open communication within the multidisciplinary team means that vital information cannot be shared (Connor et al 2010) and all members of that team are unaware of their role within the care-giving progess. Thirdly it vital to access relevant resources to ensure all decision making is evidence based. And finally, there needs to be open dialogue with the patient to make sure that they have articulated their ethical right to act with autonomy.

Overall, what is your impression of the example? How would you rate the attention to detail?

....

....

A correct version of the text is available in the feedback section. Be aware, though, that there are several ways this could have been re-drafted to make more sense.

Common mistakes in essay writing

Finally, we thought it was worth giving you the benefit of our experience. We read loads of essays, and time and again it's the same mistakes that stop people getting the marks that they would hope for. We've listed our top four errors below.

1. Failing to answer the question or address the topic fully

- Don't go off at a tangent.
- Make sure you focus on the specifics.

- Relate the topic to the role of the nurse and (more often than not) your particular field (e.g. child, mental health).
- Read the assessment guidelines through several times.

2. Too much description and no real engagement with the topic

- You will rarely (if ever) be asked to simply describe something.
- What does the information mean for nursing practice?
- Does your essay have some kind of logical flow and argument within it (think of a lawyer presenting a case)?

3. Not enough evidence or references

- There is no ideal number of texts you should read and refer to in your assessment but it should be more than ten.
- Read widely around a subject.
- Provide evidence for your statements.
- If in doubt, check that you have a reference for every fact, statistic, definition, statement or opinion.
- Be cautious in your claims (*may, could, perhaps*).
- Do not present your opinion as fact.
- Remember, placement experiences or anecdotal evidence can t be used. You need to find credible published sources.

4. No structure to the work

- The assessment should be clearly structured with signposts from one topic to the next.
- No 'stream of consciousness' writing.
- Writing a plan should help with this.

What to take from this chapter

- Write a plan. Write a plan. Write a plan!
- Think about your reader - are you leading them through your argument? Can they follow your logic?
- Think about your marker - have you given them the essay that they asked for?
- Don't run out of energy and submit something without carefully checking it.

Reflective questions

1. Will you now use an essay writing process? If so, what are the stages you will use (we suggest that there are four, but this can be adapted).

....

....

....

2. What type of plan suits your learning style? Would a mindmap plan help you visualise your argument, or would it confuse you? Try experimenting with different types of plans.

....

....

....

3. Do you need to adapt the proof-reading checklist to include your own criteria or things specific to your institution? If you can get hold of the marking guidelines, you could incorporate aspects of this into the checklist.

....

....

....

Further support

There are loads of study guides (books, websites, apps) available to help you write assessments at university. These can be a good source of advice and help boost your confidence. However, a lot of these skills are developed through practice, so don't spend so long reading the guides you run out of time to write. We would also recommend that you take advantage of all the support that your university provides.

Feedback

Activity 6.1: Your essay writing history

There's no right and wrong answer to this activity. Your observations will be completely unique to your own experiences.

Activity 6.2: An example essay

To what extent do reflective models improve the practice of healthcare professionals?

Introduction – contextual info, states what essay will cover, shows interpretation (focus on nurses)	*Reflection is the process of internally examining and exploring an issue (Boyd & Fales 1983). It involves consciously considering experiences, actions and*

feelings and then interpreting them to facilitate learning in the future (Boud et al. 1994). This essay will explore the principles of reflection and consider the importance of the concept for healthcare professionals, with particular reference to nurses. It will consider a number of reflective models and discuss the ways in which they aid nurses in becoming reflective practitioners before examining evidence to suggest that models may, in fact, inhibit the development of reflective skills.

Broad definitions of reflective practice

Reflective practice is a complex concept that has been defined in many ways (Rogers 2009, Reid 2001, Lloyd 1999). At its core, it involves practitioners learning from their experiences through the considered exploration and analysis of those events in order to inform their practice in the future. For Beattie, it is 'the mirror through which nurses can focus on themselves in a constructive, developmental manner. It allows professionals to integrate theory and reality, and work towards an ideal model of practice' (2000, p. 34).

Why reflective practice is important in healthcare

Reflective practice is considered one of the cornerstones of modern nursing (Gillies 2007). For Jacques (2005), in an ever changing social and healthcare environment, the ability of nurses to continually improve and update their practice is vital, and is enshrined in professional codes and standards (Nursing Midwifery Council (NMC 2006, NMC 2007)). Reflection is considered one of the best tools for the improvement of that practice (Livingstone 2004). In addition, Lee et al. (2010) argue that if nursing is to become the profession-alised occupation an all-degree status can afford it, it is essential practitioners engage in continuous and recordable professional development. Again, they argue that this is best achieved through reflective practice.

Outline of reflective models

A number of models exist to guide practitioners through the stages of the reflective process in a structured way (Michaels 2006). Perhaps the most commonly used within nursing (Evans & Betts 2009) is Gibbs' (1988) reflective cycle. As the name implies, this is a circular model that asks a series of questions about the incident, the practi-tioner's feelings, their analysis and, ultimately, their learning plans for the future. According to Lewis et al. (2003) one of its main strengths is that it promotes action planning in this way. Johns' (2000) model of structured reflection and Rolfe's (2001) framework for reflective practice are also frequently utilised by nurses (Michaels 2006).

Why models improve practice 1

Reflective models appear to improve the practice of nurses in a number of ways. Reflection can be a difficult skill to acquire and, according to Newark and Marine (2010), novice nurses in particular can find it difficult at first. Models provide structure and guidance as practitioners begin reflection. North London NHS Trust (2009), for example, *recommends that newly qualified student nurses develop their practice with use of Gibbs' model. They argue the guidance offered in this step by step approach 'helps nurses see the links between theory and practice, your feelings and actions' (2009, p. 45).*

Why models improve practice 2

Models are also often used to ensure that learning takes place through reflection, and so practice improves. Trout et al. (2007) argue that practitioners all too easily mistake reflection for 'indulgent navel gazing', concentrating on their feelings rather than analysing events, searching for meaning and learning for the future. Models structure reflection so that analysis and action planning are distinct phases in the process. Their use maintains the positive, learning elements of the activity (Barros 2001).

Evidence against use of models

Whilst there is a large body of evidence to suggest that reflective models improve practice, some argue that their use can have a negative impact on healthcare professionals. Lurey and Wilder (2007) call for less rigid teaching of reflection within nursing education. They argue that current models inhibit personal learning styles and often lead to mechanistic, 'box ticking' exercises rather than a genuine consideration of the nursing role. Similarly, Tupay (2003) asserts that reflective models are overused in nursing.

In conclusion ...

Activity 6.3: Careless writing

Spelling: There are a lot of spelling mistakes in the extract. They are probably not due to spelling problems, but a lack of attention and time. It makes the writing look sloppy, and you may, as a result, be less interested in what the writer has to say.

Grammar and punctuation: Again, this seems rushed. There are full stops, and even words, missing. Some sentences aren't sentences.

Clarity of writing style: The poor spelling and punctuation lead to a lack of clarity. It's not obvious what the writer means.

Formality of writing style: The writer uses 'we', which is inappropriate in academic work. Otherwise, on the whole, the extract is reasonably formal.

Original text:

There are threee important aspects to clinical decision making requires three things. Firstly, practitioners should have an up date knowledge or practice int their area expertise (Smith 2008). We can then be sure that they have all the information they need to deliver appropriate care to a specific client group Secondly clear and open communication within the multidisciplinary team means that vital information cannot be shared (Connor et al 2010) and all members of that team are unaware of their role within the care-giving progess. Thirdly it vital to access relevant resources to ensure all decision making is evidence based. And finally, there needs to be open dialogue with the patient to make sure that they have articulated their ethical right to act with autonomy.

One possible revision:

There are four important aspects to clinical decision making. Firstly, practitioners should have an up-to-date knowledge of best practice in their area of expertise (Smith 2008). This should enable them to have all the information needed to deliver appropriate care to a specific client group. Secondly, clear and open communication within the multidisciplinary team allows for vital information to be shared (Connor et al. 2010), and each team member to be aware of their role within the caregiving process. Thirdly, it is vital to access relevant resources to ensure all decision making is evidence based (James 2007). Finally, there needs to be open dialogue with the patient to make sure that they have articulated their ethical right to act with autonomy.

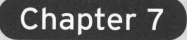

Chapter 7

Getting ready for exams

'One of my greatest fears about the degree was having to sit exams. During the first term, I put off thinking about them until the last minute, and failed. But preparing for the resit showed me how important it is to plan and put the work in.'

Second-year learning disability nursing student

LEARNING OUTCOMES

By the end of this chapter you should be able to:

● Identify three active revision methods that suit your learning style

● Apply a revision process to any upcoming exams

● Devise an action plan to cope with exam nerves

Introduction

As well as producing written work at university, you are likely to be tested under exam conditions. This chapter looks at the importance of revision planning and having a clear strategy for tackling exam questions. We also consider the potential impact of nerves on performance.

Examining exams

Many students find the prospect of exams stressful (although some people thrive on the pressure). You may not have sat any for a very long time and you may have unpleasant memories of massive exam halls and a tense atmosphere. However, they tend to be part of university life. It may be that you have to sit an exam at the end of one of your modules. Or, perhaps, it's a class test part way through. You may even have regular numeracy tests. They may all involve slightly different formats, and some may feel more serious than others, but they require similar skills. You need to recall information from memory and demonstrate your knowledge there and then.

Although they're often disliked, exams are not without their advantages. For a start, once they're over, they really are over. There is nothing you can do about your exam script once it's handed in. So you can take a deep breath and move on. Whereas with an essay you could read it through one more time, do that tiny bit more research, add that extra reference. Exams are also a really effective way of demonstrating what you know.

A lot of students tell us they find exam situations very artificial and we can definitely sympathise. In everyday life, you are rarely required to spend two hours, in complete silence, writing everything you know about a particular topic. But there are still parallels. In the clinical area, you often have to recall information quickly or communicate your intended action to others. If you think about it, this involves the same skills as drawing on your knowledge during an exam. We also increasingly hear of our graduates being asked to produce written responses to questions during interviews. Again, this sounds pretty similar to exams to us.

Basically, what we're trying to say is that, love them or loathe them, exams are likely to be part of your university experience. The good news is that, as with all other academic skills, there is plenty you can do to prepare and to develop in advance.

Revision techniques

If you have an exam or test within your course, it's really important that you don't simply assume you'll have done all the necessary learning within class and through your written work. You will need to prepare for the exams – you have to revise. Or, in some cases, you'll need to learn the content from scratch, then revise to make sure it's gone in.

There are loads of different ways to revise. You might reread your lecture notes, make a mindmap or watch documentaries on a relevant subject. Some methods are more effective than others, and as we've said elsewhere, it's important to know what works for you. Vary the way you revise. Experiment with as many methods as you can come up with. Incorporate lots of learning styles. Changing how you approach revision will help keep topics interesting and stop you getting bored.

A note on active vs passive revision

As we've already said in relation to note-taking and reading, it's possible to spend a lot of time revising without achieving anything. This happens when you're being passive – you're not interacting with the material or engaging your brain. So if you're reading a text book without taking notes or copying out a handout over and over, you're probably being passive. You need to make links, ask yourself questions or consider why something may be the case to ensure that you're being active. You need to actually do something with the content.

The easy way to tell is to ask yourself what the lazy part of you would prefer to do, and then ignore it. It's just time wasted. You're better off spending twenty concentrated minutes on a mindmap than staring at a book distractedly for an hour.

ACTIVITY 7.1: ACTIVE REVISION STRATEGIES

Think of as many different ways of revising as possible. Which do you typically use? How can you make them as active as possible? Complete the table below.

Revision strategy	Used it effectively in the past?	Active or passive?	How can it be made more active?	Suited to a particular kind of exam?
Reading over lecture notes	It's what I usually do	Passive	Summarise the notes on to ever smaller bits of paper	Good for memorising

Figure 7.1 Active revision strategies

Turn to the feedback section at the end of this chapter to read our comments.

The revision process

So you know you have a class test in eight weeks. What do you do? How do you begin preparing for it? As with essay writing, we think that revision is a process. It can begin as soon as you know when your exam or class test will take place. This means that you can plan for it, feel in control and take away that big fear of the unknown.

The process involves a number of steps:

A. Figure out **what** you are going to be tested on, i.e. what you have to revise.

B. Decide **how** you are going to do the revision: the methods you'll use.

C. Plan **when** you'll be able to revise, and make sure it's flexible enough to fit in with your life.

D. Check **if** you've been successful – so test yourself to ensure you've learned what it was you were revising.

By the time you have completed step D, you'll know which topics and issues you fully understand and have committed to memory, and which still need a bit of work. You begin the process again. But now you already

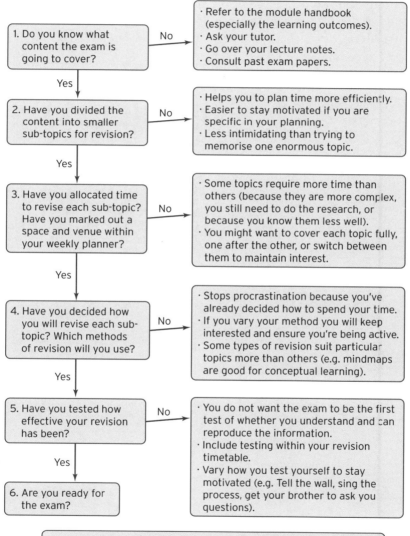

Figure 7.2 The revision process

have the answer to A – it's all the stuff you're still not sure of. You may go through several cycles before you feel fully prepared for the exam.

Another way of understanding this process is to ask yourself a series of questions.

Here's one student's use of the process. Suzie is in her third year and will shortly be sitting an exam for the module 'Care of adults with complex needs'.

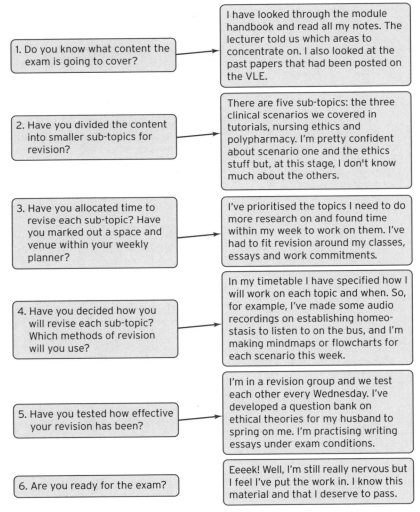

1. Do you know what content the exam is going to cover?

I have looked through the module handbook and read all my notes. The lecturer told us which areas to concentrate on. I also looked at the past papers that had been posted on the VLE.

2. Have you divided the content into smaller sub-topics for revision?

There are five sub-topics: the three clinical scenarios we covered in tutorials, nursing ethics and polypharmacy. I'm pretty confident about scenario one and the ethics stuff but, at this stage, I don't know much about the others.

3. Have you allocated time to revise each sub-topic? Have you marked out a space and venue within your weekly planner?

I've prioritised the topics I need to do more research on and found time within my week to work on them. I've had to fit revision around my classes, essays and work commitments.

4. Have you decided how you will revise each sub-topic? Which methods of revision will you use?

In my timetable I have specified how I will work on each topic and when. So, for example, I've made some audio recordings on establishing homeo-stasis to listen to on the bus, and I'm making mindmaps or flowcharts for each scenario this week.

5. Have you tested how effective your revision has been?

I'm in a revision group and we test each other every Wednesday. I've developed a question bank on ethical theories for my husband to spring on me. I'm practising writing essays under exam conditions.

6. Are you ready for the exam?

Eeeek! Well, I'm still really nervous but I feel I've put the work in. I know this material and that I deserve to pass.

Figure 7.3 Suzie's revision process

Time	Monday	Tuesday	Wednesday	Thursday	Friday	Saturday	Sunday
8.00 – 9.00	Make index card notes on communication skills		Listen to recording on bus (ipod)	Listen to recording on bus			
9.00 – 10.00		Make notes on reading for next scenario class				Take Gran to shops	Do reading for nursing studies project
10.00 – 11.00			Lecture	Clinical skills session			
11.00 – 12.00	Tutorial						
12.00 – 13.00		Lunch with Sue				Create mind map for scenario 2	
13.00 – 14.00			Tutorial				
14.00 – 15.00	Lecture			Tutorial			Cinema with Mum
15.00 – 16.00	Record explanation of nursing interventions to establish homeostasis		Meet study group in Library to divide up revision tasks for next week				
16.00 – 17.00		Babysitting niece					
17.00 – 18.00				Shift at work	Shift at work	Birthday night out for David	
18.00 – 19.00	Gym		Gym				
19.00 – 20.00							
20.00 – 21.00							

Figure 7.4 Suzie's revision timetable

Thinking about revision as a process means that you can plan well in advance. That could be setting aside a couple of hours each week for extra reading for revision notes, to a much more detailed weekly planner as you get closer to the exam date.

Go to our companion website to access blank revision planning templates.

Memory

Sometimes your revision requires you to build an argument, to understand the logical flow of a theory, for example. Other times it's purely about recalling information, such as correctly labelling a diagram of the human heart. Knowing how your memory works and creating memory triggers will help with both, but especially the latter.

ACTIVITY 7.2: HOW *YOUR* MEMORY WORKS

1. Make a note of a significant childhood event. It could be happy, sad – anything at all, so long as you can remember it very clearly.

....

....

How did you recall the detail? Do you associate the memory with any particular smells (canteen food, your gran's perfume)? Do you visually replay the scenes in your head (kind of like watching it on TV)? Is it sounds and voices that stick out to you? Or, is it more emotional – how you felt at that time?

....

....

Memory is very powerful, and we make lots of connections and associations in our mind, often without realising. How can you use this knowledge to revise and help make triggers for your memories?

....

....

2. Now think about an advert that you can't get out of your head once you've seen it. What is it that makes it so powerful? A jingle, bright colours or a cheesy slogan? A catchphrase or brand? The sheer oddness of it?

....

....

Can any of this be used in your revision? Can you put together a slogan or find another creative way to recall information?

....

....

Turn to the feedback section at the end of this chapter to read our comments.

Try not to learn 'facts' or information in isolation. Our brains don't work well that way and, for nursing, it's important to be able to put details into context. You are learning the content that you are in order to provide care to patients. So you need to be able to use that learning, apply it to practice, make links with real life. When you are revising, try to make connections between pieces of information and see the bigger picture. This will help you to memorise and recall details within exams but also helps your nursing in general.

Exam strategies

As well as revising, you have to think about how you'll actually approach the exam. For oral and clinical skills exams you'll obviously have to practise lots. For written exams, it's more about planning your time within them.

> ## A note on preparation
>
> The more you can know about the exam in advance, the better. This will help you to be prepared and feel in control. So, know the time and the venue – even visit it beforehand so you know how to get there and can visualise the layout. Make sure you have all the equipment you need (pens, etc.) and a few spares. Try to get a good night's sleep and eat something before you go, but don't beat yourself up if you're too nervous to.

We think there are three key features to developing an effective written exam strategy:

1. Planning

- Examine the whole paper and understand the instructions.
- Plan your strategy – which questions, how many marks?
- Plan your answers.

2. Timing

- Allocate time for reading the whole question paper.
- Leave time at the end to check your answers.
- Work out how long you can spend on each answer (use mark allocation) and stick to it.

3. Answering the question

- Spend time analysing the question.
- What exactly are you being asked?
- Do not write everything you know about the general subject. Answer the question.

Remember, *you* are in charge. It's *your* opportunity to demonstrate what you know. You can choose the order in which you answer questions. You can use as much paper as you need. You can cross out mistakes, take out entire sections if you like. Take control.

Types of exam questions

It's worth trying to find out about the format of the exam in advance. Is it an open-book exam (one in which you can take your text books with you)? Do you have a choice of questions? How are the marks distributed? The more you know the more you can plan.

Typically, exam questions fall into a few categories. You'll take a different approach to each. The most common are:

Multiple choice questions

A good strategy for dealing with multiple choice questions is to use a process of elimination – take away the answers that you know are wrong. Read the question very carefully – 'which is the *least* likely', 'which is the *most* likely'. Usually, we would advise you to go with your instinct if you are unsure. But make sure there is no negative marking (where you get marks deducted for choosing the wrong answer). If there is, you may only want to answer when you are fairly certain of the right response. And finally, use your time effectively – don't get stuck on one question. Note the number and come back to it.

Short answer questions

Short answer questions don't tend to ask for much detail. You can often use the number of marks on offer as a guide to how many points you should be making in your answer. Unless you're told otherwise, make sure you give full answers and use proper sentences.

Long answer/essay questions

These tend to be worth a lot of marks, and are like small essays. So start off by analysing the question. What's the topic? What's the focus? Try not to simply write everything you know about a subject. Think carefully about your structure. Plan your answer (even if you score this out later) and make sure you have a beginning, middle and end. Is there a logical progression to your argument?

Obviously, in exam conditions, you have time constraints, so you won't have forever to plan. Leave space for the answers that might occur to you part of the way through the exam. If you can only remember two of the three issues, for example, begin with those and come back to the third later.

Again, as with essays, it's important to leave time for proof-reading, so give yourself five minutes or so to go over your answer. It's amazing the kinds of simple mistakes that you can make under pressure. These are easily corrected if you allow time for a final read through.

 Go to our companion website to try an online activity on exam questions and planning.

Coping with nerves

Do you get nervous before an exam? Does your anxiety affect your performance?

A little adrenaline is a good thing – it will help you concentrate and stay alert during the exam. Nerves are perfectly natural and most of us

	A few months/ weeks before	A few days before	During the exam
How nerves might affect you	Ostrich syndrome (sticking your head in the sand). Building up the exams into a bigger thing than they really are.	Use up what little time you have panicking. Flit from topic to topic without learning anything. Spend hours on passive revision.	Panic, forget information you know you know. Misread questions or instructions. Waste time.
What you can do	Try hypnotherapy or relaxation techniques. Begin your preparation: write a revision plan. Confront your fears (do some mock exams).	Prioritise (what topics, how long, when?). Use your time wisely but make sure you get some rest. Test yourself.	Regulate your breathing. Prepare some relaxation techniques. Begin with what you do know.

Figure 7.5 Exam nerves timeline

experience them, but too many and they could get in the way of your success.

If you are very worried about upcoming exams, it is probably best that you start to develop coping strategies straight away.

Worst case scenarios

We talk to a lot of worriers. Despite all the preparation, students still fear that the worst is going to happen. Here's our advice:

Scenario 1: My mind goes blank!

1. Recognise this is a normal response to stress and it is temporary.
2. Breathe. It's easy to forget to do this.
3. Choose a question if you have not already.
4. Think what an answer should look like. Recall your 'triggers'.
5. If you are still blank, think back to your course – the lectures, classes, placements. Picture the lecturer speaking or visualise the textbook.
6. Focus your mind with basic questions: **What** is the main issue? **Where** is this case? **Why** does it happen?
7. Note down any ideas that come to mind.

Scenario 2: I didn't revise any of these topics!

1. Plan ahead so this does not happen.
2. Think of ways to relate what you do know to the questions.
3. Make an argument based on the knowledge you have.
4. Better to write something than leave a question blank.

Scenario 3: I break my leg on the way to the exam!

1. Don't panic.
2. Your university will have a system in place to deal with this kind of emergency.

3. Contact the university as soon as possible.

4. Find out what the procedure is in advance, just in case.

Scenario 4: What if I fail?

There are usually opportunities to retake assessments. These are often called resits.

Resits

Nobody wants to fail. At university, when you have a lot at stake, it can be really crushing to realise that you have not passed an assessment. However, it needn't be the end of the world. In the vast majority of cases, you will have the chance to redo the assessment. Sometimes, you wait until the following summer and sit the exam again. Other times, you can retake it much sooner. It really depends on what exactly you failed and the way your particular institution works. We normally think about resits in relation to exams. But, of course, it is possible to fail any assessment. Here again though, you are likely to have the opportunity to rewrite any essay or redo any presentation that hasn't come up to scratch.

If you think about it (and we know this is easy to say), failing something can be a really good learning opportunity.

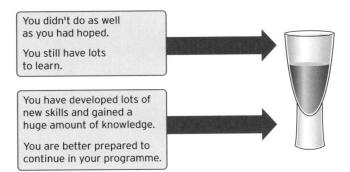

Figure 7.6 Resits - the glass half full

When we fail something, we can consider our emotional response to that, leading to personal development and, perhaps, a new outlook. We can work out what went wrong. And that provides an opportunity to work on skills, motivations and behaviours. Finally, we can put in the effort to fix the problem, which should lead to greater confidence and a sense of pride. If it's an academic failure, when we do eventually pass the assessment, we know the subject really well

Consider these two students:

Rebecca did some revision for her exam but it was the minimum she thought she could get away with. Out of the three main topics she only learned one of them. But Rebecca got lucky. It came up in the exam, she scraped a pass and was able to move on to the next module.	**Claire** thought that a lot of the module was just common sense. She also had strong clinical experience and presumed she could rely on that to get her through the exam. However, she lacked the details to fully answer the questions and had difficulty applying theories to practice issues. She failed the module and had to retake the exam a few months later. Despite it initially knocking her confidence, Claire decided to set aside at least two hours each week to revise the material. She passed the resit well and is sure she can tackle any future exams. She is now also much more confident with the course content and her study skills.

Initially, you might think that Rebecca was the more fortunate. Everyone wants to pass first time. But it's only really of value if you actually know and understand the stuff, especially in a discipline like nursing. It's Claire who comes through the experience with stronger skills and knowledge.

Figuring out what went wrong and fixing it

The most important thing to do if you fail an assessment is spend time figuring out why. This can be quite tricky, and possibly draining, but you have to do it if you are going to pass next time round. There are several possible categories in which you may have come unstuck:

- Was it a problem with preparation? Did you plan your revision? Did you dedicate enough time to it?

- Was it something to do with skills? Do you have recall strategies? Can you compose a logical argument?

- Was it the subject content? Did you understand the material and theory? Did you do enough reading?

- Was there an issue with your lifestyle? Too many late nights? Too much worrying?

- Were there any other barriers? Child-care issues? Part-time work taking up too much time?

It's important to take an honest look at what happened. It's your responsibility as an independent learner. But, equally, there's little point in giving yourself a hard time for something that's in the past. Choose to do something constructive and pinpoint the difficult area rather than deciding that you are entirely useless.

 Go to our companion website to take the 'what went wrong' quiz. This is probably of most use if you have a resit to do.

As well as personally reflecting on what went wrong, it's vital you speak to academic staff. Ask for feedback (we cover this later), find out why you received the mark (grade) you did and get advice on tackling the resit. It's unlikely you're the only one in that situation and staff do want you to pass. Once you have all of this information you can devise a plan of revision and skills development so that you pass next time round. Remember, investing time and effort now will not only help with the resit, but all future assessments.

Handling feedback

What is it?

It is common to receive feedback on all types of academic work. It can come in many different forms:

- verbal feedback from academic staff or fellow students
- written comments from your tutor accompanying your mark
- one-to-one discussion with your tutor
- pre-prepared statements on a feedback form
- with exams you may not receive much feedback apart from your mark but you can ask for more information.

Why should I care?

Inevitably, your main concern is your mark – did I pass or fail?

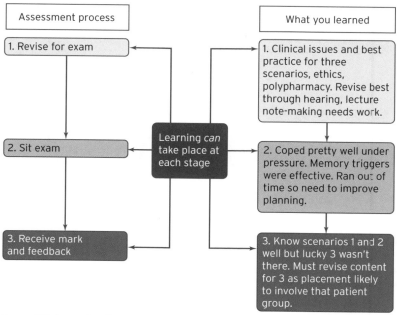

Figure 7.7 Learning from exam feedback

But, it is really important you look beyond that, to the feedback you are given:

- It tells you *why* you received the mark you did.
- It will highlight the positives of your work.
- It lets you know where you need to improve (e.g. referencing, providing more supporting evidence).

Even if you have passed an assessment, or have done really well, it's still best to spend time considering the feedback you have been given. It's a large part of the learning process.

The same is true for essays, or any other assessment. You can learn as much by engaging with the feedback as you can from the initial research.

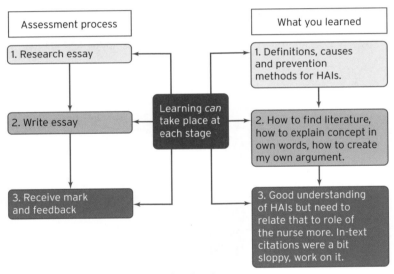

Figure 7.8 Learning from essay feedback

How do I use it?

- Try not to react emotionally – don't get angry, upset or defensive. Maybe give yourself a bit of time to get over your initial feelings. Then read the comments again in as objective a way as you can.

- Reread your assessment and try to see the areas mentioned in the comments.

- Categorise feedback into different areas – e.g. finding resources, referencing, writing style.

- Draw up an action plan to work on any weaknesses.

- Is there anything you don't understand? If so, make an appointment with your tutor to discuss it. Don't be worried about looking silly. Tutors give feedback so you can learn. They expect you to talk to them about it.

- Read over past feedback before submitting any work. This will help you spot any errors you are prone to making.

What to take from this chapter

- Exams can be stressful and people can really dislike them, but it is possible to take control, and that can have a huge impact on your confidence.

- Keep your revision active. Check if you are paying attention, and continually test how effective your revision has been.

- Find out what you can beforehand. Know what to expect in terms of content, format, location, marking. Don't be afraid to ask for information on these things. Ask for feedback on your performance afterwards.

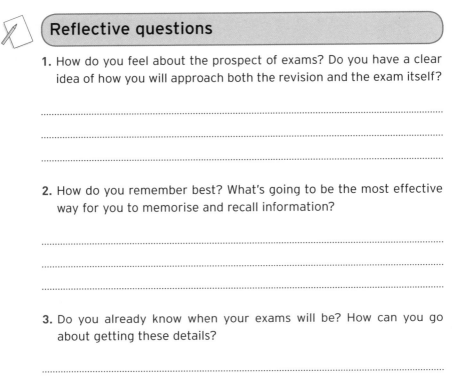

Reflective questions

1. How do you feel about the prospect of exams? Do you have a clear idea of how you will approach both the revision and the exam itself?

....

....

....

2. How do you remember best? What's going to be the most effective way for you to memorise and recall information?

....

....

....

3. Do you already know when your exams will be? How can you go about getting these details?

....

....

....

Further support

As with other academic skills, there are lots of study guides and websites on exam skills.

Weyers, J. and McMillan, K. (2011). *How to Succeed in Exams and Assessments*, Pearson Education Ltd.

There is also lots of advice available online, specifically for students, about coping with exam nerves. The mental health charity MIND has a particularly good page:

http://www.mind.org.uk/help/diagnoses_and_conditions/exam_stress

Feedback

Activity 7.1: Active revision strategies

Here are some suggestions of different ways to actively revise:

- Summarise your notes onto index cards.
- Put stickers with revision material all over your house. You could even use a different room for each topic.
- Use colours, songs and smells to help you remember things.
- Explain an idea to someone – it helps you to check you really understand something.
- Write essay questions and plan your answers.
- Get friends or family to test you.
- Try answering questions from past papers.
- Create mindmaps.
- Time yourself under mock exam conditions.
- Set up a revision study group.
- Record yourself giving an explanation of a topic.
- Ask your tutor for a practice exam.
- Go over an argument in your head while exercising or doing the dishes.
- Give yourself ten minutes to read and record as much of a book chapter as you can and then test yourself.
- Practise drawing diagrams from memory.
- Create a bank of multiple choice questions.

Activity 7.2: How *your* memory works

1. We use lots of methods to recall information, and it is surprising how strong some of the more unusual associations can be. Think about using sights, sounds or smells to create triggers and retrieve information in exam conditions. If your memories are particularly driven by emotions and how you feel, for example, can you draw on placement experiences? Or can you remember where the lecture

on a particular subject took place? The more routes you can find to recalling information, the better the chance you have of doing so.

2. Advertisers are brilliant at making things unforgettable. Again, it's all about the triggers. You hear those three notes, and you're already singing the rest of the tune. Try to incorporate triggers into your revision.

Chapter 8

Getting ready for other assessments

'I really like that it isn't all essays on my course. Sometimes we do exams at the end of a module, other times we give a presentation or take part in a clinical assessment. If you aren't so good in one, you tend to be able to make up for it in another'.

Second-year learning disability nursing student

LEARNING OUTCOMES

By the end of this chapter you should be able to:

- Describe the purpose and features of reflective writing
- Plan and confidently deliver a presentation
- Identify ways to effectively participate in group work

Introduction

There are many ways that you may be assessed on your course, other than through pieces of written academic work and exams. In this chapter we'll look at reflective assessments, presentations and group work.

Reflective assessments

What is reflection?

Nurses use reflection to evaluate and improve their practice. It's a way of thinking about what you do as a nurse and why: if a particular action has been effective; how you felt about a scenario; if your practice is based on evidence; what you might do differently next time. Nurses don't do what they do just because it's always been like that or because a superior told them to. But how can they become aware of what they're doing and judge it? Well, that's where reflection comes in.

Reflection is about learning from your experiences to improve your nursing.

ACTIVITY 8.1: A ROUGH AND READY EXERCISE ON REFLECTION

Write a list of three things you have done in the past week that are different from what you would usually do (this could be taking the bus instead of the train or talking to someone new, for example). Beside each one write down the information or skills that you already had which helped you know what to do. Ask yourself how and why you did what you did, and then think about other ways that you could have approached the action, and how you might do things differently in the future.

	What did you do?	What info?	What skills?	Would you do anything differently?
1.				
2.				
3.				

Figure 8.1 Exercise on reflection

Turn to the feedback section at the end of this chapter to read our comments.

What are reflective assessments?

We think about what we're doing all the time: what it means, how it feels, if it worked. So that means that we tend to have the basic skills for reflection already. But the reflective process is much more considered and structured than everyday musings. In fact, it's likely to be a feature of your assessments at university. You'll demonstrate your learning through reflective diaries, essays or action plans for the future.

A note on critical incidents

Anything that happens to us or anything we do on a daily basis can be reflected upon. In your studies and in your professional life, however, you will probably reflect on particularly *significant* events. It could be significant because of the implications, because of the effect on your learning or because of the strength of your feelings. It's likely that these will be referred to as *critical incidents*.

Reflection is often considered to be about identifying and addressing your weaknesses, but a critical incident could just as easily focus on something that you've done well. Reflection should be about your strengths too.

Choose the incident you want to reflect on with care. You need to be comfortable talking about it and there should be sufficient scope for discussion and analysis.

You'll be introduced to different models of reflection during your degree. Though they'll vary slightly, their basic aim is the same – to help you engage in the structured process of reflection. This involves a number of steps:

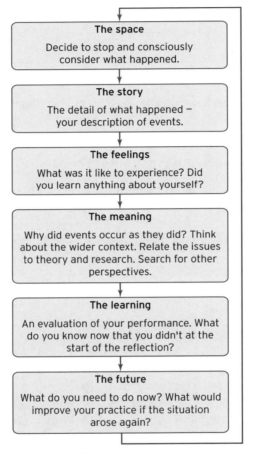

Figure 8.2 Understanding reflection as a process

To help you understand how you might go through the reflective process, we've provided an example of a student's reflective notes. We've added some comments about common mistakes that we often see during this process.

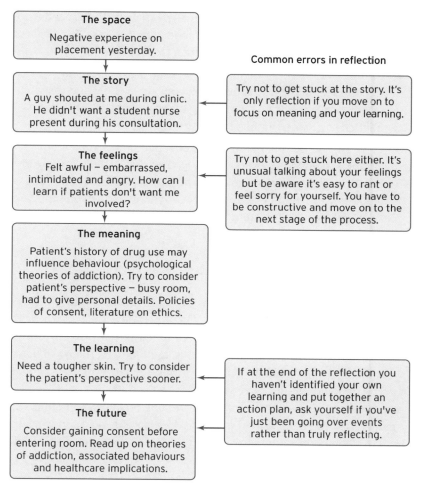

The space
Negative experience on placement yesterday.

Common errors in reflection

The story
A guy shouted at me during clinic. He didn't want a student nurse present during his consultation.

Try not to get stuck at the story. It's only reflection if you move on to focus on meaning and your learning.

The feelings
Felt awful – embarrassed, intimidated and angry. How can I learn if patients don't want me involved?

Try not to get stuck here either. It's unusual talking about your feelings but be aware it's easy to rant or feel sorry for yourself. You have to be constructive and move on to the next stage of the process.

The meaning
Patient's history of drug use may influence behaviour (psychological theories of addiction). Try to consider patient's perspective – busy room, had to give personal details. Policies of consent, literature on ethics.

The learning
Need a tougher skin. Try to consider the patient's perspective sooner.

If at the end of the reflection you haven't identified your own learning and put together an action plan, ask yourself if you've just been going over events rather than truly reflecting.

The future
Consider gaining consent before entering room. Read up on theories of addiction, associated behaviours and healthcare implications.

Figure 8.3 Example of reflective notes and common errors

Why do I need to reflect?

Reflection *will* be a feature of your degree as it's such a big part of nursing.

● It helps practitioners to link theory and practice. There are all the things you learn at university and through your reading, and then there are all the things that happen on placement. Sometimes the connection is clear – a lecture on wound dressing will provide you with information for when you actually carry out the procedure. But often, the link isn't quite so immediately obvious. The process of reflection consciously brings those two spheres together.

- It's a way of problem solving for everyday practice. Again, reflection allows you to draw on all your theoretical and research-based knowledge. It lets you analyse and evaluate your routine practice to ensure that it's the best it can be.

- As we've said before, nursing is a reflective profession. You'll continue to engage in it long after you've graduated. So think of it less as a skill you'll need solely for university than one that you'll need for your lifelong career. In fact, if you engage in any further study once you're registered, you're likely to be assessed through reflective work.

Features of reflective writing

Reflection is a thinking task, but it's often documented by way of writing. For assessments, you will almost certainly reflect in a written form. Whilst you might be disheartened to learn that reflective writing is distinctive, with some of its own rules and features, the good news is that it still shares much in common with academic writing.

The defining feature of reflective writing is that it's about you: your experiences; your learning; often even your feelings. Sometimes this means that you'll be writing in the first person (using 'I') in work that you're handing in to be assessed. As with all the other skills, this will take a bit of practice and development.

	Reflective	Academic
Uses 'I' and personal experience	✓	✗
Is formal (not a diary or a blog)	✓	✓
Has a clear structure (intro, main body, conclusion)	✓	✓
Includes evidence and references	✓	✓
Considers other perspectives and looks for meaning	✓	✓
Clearly shows what you've learned	✓	✗

Figure 8.4 Features of reflective and academic writing

You wouldn't necessarily expect something that you write about yourself to include an introduction, main body and conclusion or to have references, but as we've outlined above, it does. Consider the examples in the following activity.

ACTIVITY 8.2: EXTRACTS OF REFLECTIVE WRITING

Here are three extracts which reflect on the same critical incident. What comments do you have on each of the extracts? Are they reflective?

Extract 1

> *On my third day in the ward, I was asked to assist with Mr X's bathing. He was admitted after a fall last week and remains unsteady on his feet. Normally he lives at home with his wife, who has been his primary carer since he was diagnosed with dementia three years ago.*
>
> *I had chatted with Mr X on a previous occasion during drugs rounds, but had not spent much time with him. As soon as I began to bathe him I realised that I was unable to communicate with him very effectively. I wasn't sure if he understood me, and couldn't tell if he was uncomfortable being bathed by a young, female student nurse. However, I tried to be as professional as possible.*

....

....

....

Extract 2

> *Today I had to bathe an elderly, male patient. I found the experience really mortifying and can't believe I was put in that position by my mentor. I was so embarrassed I found it impossible to start a conversation and tried not to make eye contact. I don't plan on working with the elderly when I register, so I don't see what good this experience has done me.*

....

....

....

Extract 3

> *It became clear when bathing Mr X that I was not able to understand his vocalisations and couldn't determine whether he knew what I was saying. Cartwright (2009) has suggested that there may be significant challenges in communicating with dementia patients. This raises issues of consent (Gallen 2008), and the nurse's role in ensuring respect for patients (NMC 2010). I had no way of knowing whether my actions were clear and consented to.*
>
> *I plan to research theories of communication and effective strategies for use with dementia patients to improve my ability to care for Mr X.*

....

....

....

Turn to the feedback section at the end of this chapter to read our comments.

If it seems a bit exasperating that this seems to be a whole new way of writing, remember that there are some really great things about reflection. Our students often get frustrated that there is nothing of themselves in their assessments. Reflective work is all about you, your learning and your experiences. It also concerns the reality of the nursing profession.

Presentations

Over the course of your degree it's highly likely that you will be expected to give a presentation in some form or other. It may be as part of a group during a problem-based learning tutorial, it may be as an individual to your tutor group. You might need to deliver it alongside a slideshow presentation or it may involve giving a quick overview of a topic and then answering questions. Sometimes, you get to create a large poster that contains all of the information. You then present a summary and receive questions while standing by your poster.

While some people are natural-born performers, many of us are uncomfortable with the idea of speaking in public. But, as with all other skills we've talked about, we believe there's lots you can do to improve your abilities and confidence.

The good, the bad and the ugly of presentations

However you feel about presentations, it's worth considering why they are part of your degree. They have real positives for students in terms of development and experience for the future.

Presentation positives	Presentation negatives
They are a chance to demonstrate your knowledge.	The very thought of them can make people nervous. This can actually have an impact on your performance.
Presenting is now part of professional life so there's basically no escaping it. You'll need presentation skills in shift handovers, for further courses, and even in getting the job in the first place.	Public speaking may be a very new skill to you. It's often something people avoid.
They provide an opportunity to ask for others' opinions. Feedback and questions afterwards can often really improve your learning and your confidence.	Students can be worried about the reaction of their audience. Will they be listened to? Will people laugh? As the presenter you have the right to expect the audience's attention and respect. At university, you can be confident this will be the case (it's likely your fellow students will have to take their turn and you can trust staff to create a supportive atmosphere).
They encourage you to try new media. You could use video or audio clips to get your point across. You could learn to use new software (OpenOffice Impress, Microsoft PowerPoint, for example).	Presentations often involve technology and this can create anxiety (I don't know how to move the slide on. I don't know how to use this software).
They help you develop the ability to convey often complex information to a specific audience. This is a vital nursing skill when communicating with patients.	Your time to do the presentation will be limited. You frequently have to deliver a lot of detailed information in a short space of time. This is tricky.

![thumbs up] Presentation positives	![thumbs down] Presentation negatives
Presentations can really suit some people's learning styles/preferences. Students often tell us they can explain a concept really well, they just can't write it down. Well, this is their chance.	
They require and develop skills that you use elsewhere in your degree, such as researching information and evidence or planning and building an argument.	
They draw on your creative skills. Often you have a lot more flexibility in design than you do with an essay, for example.	

Figure 8.5 The positives and negatives of presentations

A good presentation guide: the checklists

To receive a good mark for a presentation assessment you need to consider four key areas.

1. Planning

As with all work, preparation and planning are essential. You have to know what is expected and actually put the hours in. Do you fully understand the assessment guidelines for a start?

2. Getting content

Once you know the details of your assessment, you need to figure out what you are actually going to say. As with any written work or exam, you will be expected to gather information, conduct research and construct your argument.

Questions to consider	Answer	Action if unsure?
How will the presentation be marked?		
When and where will it take place?		
How long is it expected to last?		
Is it an individual or a group presentation?		
Am I expected to provide a slideshow and/or handouts?		
Who is the audience? At what level should I 'pitch' it?		
Will I take questions from the audience during or after?		
What equipment/software should I use?		
When do I have the time to work on it?		
Where will I get the content from?		
When will I rehearse?		

Figure 8.6 The presentation planning checklist

Questions to consider	Answer	Action if unsure?
Have I devised a plan and thought about structure?		
Have I done sufficient reading?		
Is my evidence credible and up to date?		
Does my introduction set the scene and say what's to come?		
Do I lead the audience through the argument logically?		
Have I considered the implications and related them to nursing?		
Do I summarise my main points at the end?		
Do I provide references on my slides/handout?		
Should I provide questions to get the audience thinking?		
Is my background knowledge enough to take questions?		
Would any props, media, examples add clarity?		

Figure 8.7 The presentation content checklist

3. The technicalities

It's probable you'll accompany your presentation with supporting slides, a poster or, at the very least, a handout. This is often a really good way of guiding your delivery and providing you with memory prompts. These visual aids have the advantage of keeping the audience's attention while shifting the focus away from you. There are a number of practical things you'll have to consider. For example, do the assessment guidelines give any specific advice on the layout or font you should use in slides?

Questions to consider	Answer	Action if unsure?
What technical facilities do I have available to me?		
Do I have a back-up plan if the technology fails?		
Are all slides visually clear (font, text size, spacing)?		
Are slides succinct (i.e. not too many words)?		
Are slides in a logical order for audience to follow?		
Do slides have a clear purpose without distracting?		
Are slides attractive to look at?		
Are slides consistent in appearance?		
Do slides show where evidence comes from?		
Have I practised navigating through the slideshow?		
Have I checked that links, videos etc. work in venue?		

Figure 8.8 The presentation technicalities checklist

A note on good slide vs bad slide

Presentation software can be great and using slides can really enhance a presentation. But be aware that there are a number of simple design and layout principles you should consider. It's so easy to get carried away and end up with unreadable or distracting slides.

- Far too much text
- Image unrelated to content
- Choice of colours makes text unreadable
- Spelling mistake
- Font style and size unhelpful

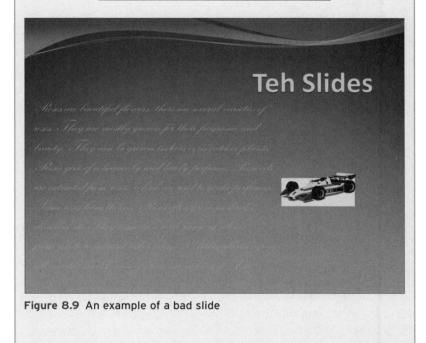

Figure 8.9 An example of a bad slide

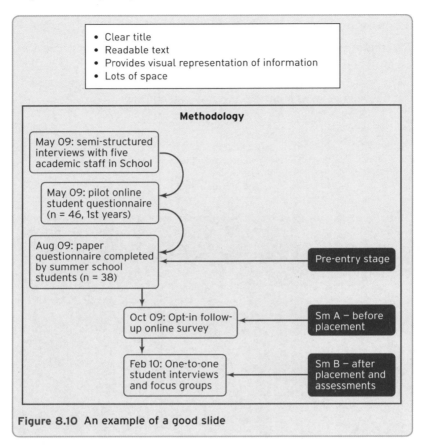

Figure 8.10 An example of a good slide

4. The delivery

Of course, the biggest part of the presentation is actually delivering it. Having been through the previous three stages you should be in a really good position to give your talk. However, you also need to be prepared for the day itself. There are things you can do that will help combat any nerves, enhance your performance and make sure things go smoothly.

Questions to consider	Answer	Action if unsure?
Am I speaking in a varied tone to maintain interest?		
Am I speaking too quickly or in too high a pitch?		
What image am I projecting – confident, enthusiastic?		
Am I waving my hands about too much?		
Am I making sufficient eye contact with the audience?		
Am I only using notes as a prompt?		
Have I practised enough to know it inside out?		
Do I know timings – when I should be at what point?		
If in a group, have we practised changeovers?		
Can I pronounce everything correctly?		
Have I included breathing breaks (quick drink)?		
Have I prepared last sentence to indicate the finish?		

Figure 8.11 The presentation delivery checklist

 Go to our companion website to view some examples of presentations.

Presentations can be challenging but if you've done the preparation, had sufficient run-throughs and are confident with the material, there's no reason you shouldn't do well. No one knows how you are feeling, so if you are wracked with nerves, just fake it.

Group work

Group work in assessments

Group work is a common feature of learning at university. You'll be studying alongside other students in lots of different contexts: in tutorials, on placement and as part of problem based learning. You may even set up your own study or revision groups to share tasks and keep each other motivated. So, whilst you're an independent learner at university, you're not an isolated learner.

You also sometimes participate in group work that is assessed. For example:

- As a group of four you may have to research and develop a presentation on the effects of social class on health.

- In pairs, you might have to find and evaluate a journal paper on chronic obstructive pulmonary disease (COPD). You could be expected to share the main points with your tutorial group.

- You and seven other students might be asked to devise a health promotion campaign for young pregnant smokers. Your assessment could be to pitch the campaign to prospective funders.

Group work can be fun in and of itself, but it's not without its challenges. You can sometimes be reliant on other people for your mark when you may prefer plugging away alone, or you might find splitting a task difficult. But group work is part of your degree because it allows for the development of key skills. These include clear and effective communication, negotiation, collaborative working and the opportunity to build leadership skills. You've worked in lots of groups before (as part of a family, as a team at work, in sport) so you'll have lots of these skills already.

For a nursing degree in particular, it's really important that group work is included as it's such an essential part of your professional skill set. You'll work in partnership with other nursing practitioners and as a member of inter-professional teams (i.e. with doctors, physios, dieticians, social workers).

Each group that you're part of will have a different purpose, different people with different roles and a different dynamic.

A note on roles in groups

In any group, people take on different roles. Your role will vary depending on the group, and the particular situation. Some roles are helpful, some are necessary, but some can be problematic. We're all aware of these group dynamics and behaviours on some level, because we're social animals.

Think about home, and how you and those around you slot into certain roles in certain circumstances. In a crisis, perhaps it's always the same person who steps up. When it comes to organising money, maybe it's you who always takes the lead and it can feel like others are just sitting back.

But in an academic setting you need to be more conscious of the situation. It's important that your group is working as effectively as it can. Work out what roles are needed (the practical organiser, the motivator, the techie) and what behaviours might hold the group back (bossiness, apathy, sulkiness). Try a variety of these essential roles, so you're constantly developing your skills and you know that you're taking responsibility. It's great to play to your strengths, but your degree is about developing additional ones. As a group, try to avoid behaviours that might negatively impact upon your progress.

ACTIVITY 8.3: RESOLVING GROUP WORK ISSUES

Consider these group work scenarios. What can you suggest to resolve any difficulties and successfully complete the task?

Scenario 1

A group of six students are working together on a series of problem based clinical scenarios over the course of the first semester. They have met three times so far. Two members of the group tend to have very strong opinions, and often clash. They dominate discussions, meaning other members, two in particular, remain very quiet. The group has made very little progress up until now. They're all frustrated at the lack of learning, but no one has said so.

What might improve the situation for all members of the group?

....

....

....

Scenario 2

Four students have been put into a group by their tutor. They will deliver a presentation in three weeks' time. They have divided the topic into four areas and agreed to individually research and write about one. They plan to meet up on the morning of the presentation to rehearse.

Can or should the group do anything differently?

....

....

....

Turn to the feedback section at the end of this chapter to read our comments.

Top tips on creating a successful group

1. **Establish ground rules at a very early stage.** Decide the aims of the group and agree on what is expected of all participants. In each group you're in these rules are likely to be different and will depend on the task.

2. **Make sure you keep in touch with each other.** Swap phone numbers and email addresses, for example.

3. **Be sure that everyone knows what they are supposed to be doing.** Often the easiest way of doing this is by having someone take notes on what is agreed and then distributing them to everyone in the group. It is harder for people to wriggle out of or forget their responsibilities when it is in front of them in black and white.

4. **Keep everyone informed.** If a member of your group has to miss a meeting, make sure that someone takes responsibility for contacting and updating them.

5. **Try to settle disputes.** If you do have any problems, the first thing you should do is talk to the other members of your group. Let them know what is wrong and, hopefully, you will be able to sort it out together. It can be difficult to tell people that you are having a problem with them but if you air your views calmly and with sensitivity it can be the best way of settling any dispute. Make sure you criticise ideas or behaviours rather than the person.

6. **Know where to turn in the worst case scenario.** If someone has gone AWOL or communication has totally broken down between members, then speak to staff. It's far better to handle issues between yourselves, but it's not always possible.

7. **Be aware of your own behaviour.** Are you unintentionally appearing bored? Is there anything you could do to encourage someone to contribute? Are you pulling your weight, but not taking over?

What to take from this chapter

- Remember that reflective writing is still academic. It's so easy to become chatty or write like a diary entry when you're talking about your personal experience. So don't.

- A good presentation is about what's in it as well as how it's delivered. Put the work in to make sure you're confident of the material, and practise, practise, practise.

- Recognise that group work can develop your skills for nursing, and try to take on different roles each time you participate.

Reflective questions

1. How do you feel about the prospect of reflection on your programme? Do you plan to practise beforehand?

....

....

....

2. What experiences have you had presenting in the past? What are your strengths and weaknesses regarding this type of assessment?

....

....

....

3. When have you been part of a successful team? What kind of role did you play? Why did it work so effectively?

....

....

....

Further support

Your university is likely to offer resources, and perhaps even classes and workshops, on developing presentation and group work skills. Have a look at the website, or ask if you can't find any details.

For reflection, our students find the following introductory book particularly informative:

Jasper, M. (2003). *Beginning Reflective Practice*, Nelson Thornes.

Feedback

Activity 8.1: A rough and ready exercise on reflection

	What did you do?	What info?	What skills?	Would you do anything differently?
1.	Recently began caring for two elderly cats.	Both require different foods, and one has regular medicine.	Time management (get up earlier). Planning (ensure sufficient food available).	Fit cat flaps in advance to prevent initial accidents.

Figure 8.12 Exercise on reflection – an example

Activity 8.2: Extracts of reflective writing

Comments on Extract 1

Although clearly written in a formal, academic style, this extract is purely descriptive. It tells us nothing about what the student has learned, how she felt, and what action she will take in the future. She provides good background detail, but fails to include references to locate the issues within the literature.

Comments on Extract 2

This focuses too much on the personal. There's no consideration of the patient's perspective, for example. It almost comes across as a bit of a whinge. No one's saying that you won't feel like this now and again, but it isn't what reflective writing is about.

Comments on Extract 3

This extract has a good balance. We're told about the student's experience. She looks for meaning by relating the events to relevant literature, theory and policy. The student also identifies how she will develop her knowledge and practice in the future.

Activity 8.3: Resolving group work issues

Scenario 1

There are a number of things the members could try:

- Perhaps agree to one leader or chair. This might stop the fight for control, and the chair could make sure everyone's voice was heard.

- Have rotating roles, so that everyone has an opportunity to lead and must take their share of responsibility.

- Agree that at the end of every meeting they will create a task list. This might state who will do what by the following week.

- Each member could also probably be a little more sympathetic to the feelings of the others. It's not fair to sit in silence, but it's also not right to monopolise the conversation.

Scenario 2

This isn't really group work. If they're being marked as individuals, it may not matter too much. But they'll still be missing out on the opportunity to learn from each other and develop team-working skills. To gain more from the experience, they might

- Meet up more regularly to discuss the content and their progress

- Put the presentation together as a group (check structure, avoid duplication, ensure consistency of slides)

- Leave more time for rehearsal (practise timing, give feedback on performance, agree on terminology and pronunciation)

- Topics are likely to interrelate, so group discussion would generate ideas and deeper engagement.

Index